Instant DNB Obs/Gyne Questions

By Swati Ahuja

Peepee Publishers and Distributors Private Limited®

Instant DNB Obs/gyne Questions

Published by
Pawaninder P. Vij and Anupam Vij

Peepee Publishers and Distributors Private Limited
Head Office: 160, Shakti Vihar, Pitam Pura
Delhi-110 034 (India)

Correspondence Address:

7/31, First Floor, Ansari Road, Daryaganj
New Delhi-110002 (India)

Ph: 41512412, 9811156083

e-mail: peepee160@yahoo.co.in

e-mail: peepee160@gmail.com

www.peepeepub.com

First Edition: 2024

ISBN: 978-81-9720-726-6

Preface

If you are preparing for the DNB Obstetrics and Gynecology exam and in search of reliable, comprehensive study materials, consider the "Instant DNB Obs/Gyne Questions".

- **Topic-Wise Organization**: The book is organized by topics, encompassing all questions previously asked in these subjects during past exams. This structure allows for targeted practice and a thorough review of all key areas you will encounter on the exam.
- **Up-to-Date Content**: The book incorporates the latest advancements in Obstetrics and Gynecology, ensuring that you're studying the most current and relevant information. This integration prepares you for questions on recent developments in the field.
- **Strategic Study Planning**: The book helps you formulate an effective study plan by identifying strengths and weaknesses. This allows you to allocate your study time more efficiently, focusing on areas that need more attention to enhance your overall exam readiness.

Overall, this book is an invaluable tool for DNB aspirants. Its methodical approach, combined with comprehensive past exam data and current medical updates, makes it an indispensable guide for anyone aiming to excel in their Obstetrics and Gynecology exams.

Contents

Chapter - 1

OBSTETRICS

1. Describe the treatment approach for managing Intrahepatic Cholestasis of Pregnancy in a Primigravida at 28 weeks of gestation?
2. Discuss the underlying causes and mechanisms leading to cholestasis of pregnancy, along with a comprehensive overview of its potential complications?
3. Provide an overview of the clinical presentation, diagnosis, and management of acute fatty liver of pregnancy.
4. Provide an explanation of what Cholestasis of Pregnancy is?
5. What are the diagnostic methods used to identify Obstetric Cholestasis?
6. Explore the principles and administration of intraperitoneal hyperthermic chemotherapy (IPHC) in the treatment of abdominal cancers?
7. Explain the underlying causes and pathophysiology of acute fatty liver of pregnancy?
8. What are the underlying factors contributing to jaundice development in pregnant women?
9. Explore the different causes of jaundice during pregnancy and their implications.
10. What are the distinguishing features between acute fatty liver of pregnancy and viral hepatitis?
11. What treatment strategies would you implement for a patient diagnosed with acute fatty liver of pregnancy?
12. Outline the diagnostic process and treatment strategies for managing viral hepatitis in pregnant women?

13. What are the potential conditions other than liver-related issues that could cause jaundice in pregnant individuals?
14. Provide the diagnostic criteria or evaluation process for identifying each of the potential causes of jaundice in pregnancy?
15. What treatment plan would you recommend for managing acute fatty liver of pregnancy in a patient at 34 weeks of gestation?
16. Discuss the underlying mechanisms and therapeutic strategies for Intrahepatic Cholestasis of Pregnancy?
17. What factors contribute to the development of jaundice during pregnancy?
18. What diagnostic steps would you take and what treatment approach would you recommend for a patient diagnosed with intrahepatic cholestasis of pregnancy (ICP)?
19. What potential adverse effects does intrahepatic cholestasis (IHC) pose on the fetus?
20. What factors contribute to recurrent pregnancy loss?
21. Outline the clinical management strategy for early pregnancy in individuals with anti-phospholipid antibodies (APLA).
22. How does systemic lupus erythematosus (SLE) impact pregnancy?
23. How would you approach the diagnosis and treatment of a pregnant individual with Antiphospholipid antibodies Syndrome (APLA)?
24. Systemic lupus erythematosus (SLE) and its implications during pregnancy.
25. Discuss the potential factors contributing to recurrent pregnancy loss?
26. What diagnostic steps would you take for a non-pregnant woman who has experienced three miscarriages?
27. What management strategies would you outline for a pregnant woman with a history of three intrauterine deaths at term?
28. What is meant by recurrent pregnancy loss?
29. What factors contribute to recurrent pregnancy loss (RPL)?
30. What diagnostic steps would you take in evaluating a case of recurrent pregnancy loss?

31. What are the potential factors leading to second-trimester pregnancy loss?

32. What diagnostic approach would you employ for evaluating a case of recurrent second-trimester pregnancy loss, and how would you discuss the prognosis with the patient regarding the likelihood of future occurrences in subsequent pregnancies?

33. Explain the role of anti-phospholipid antibodies in autoimmune diseases.

34. What are the clinical and laboratory criteria used to diagnose anti-phospholipid syndrome (APS)?

35. Describe the pregnancy complications linked with thrombo-philic disorders.

36. Define "bad obstetric history" (BOH) in the context of reproductive health.

37. What investigative approaches would you employ during the interval phase and throughout pregnancy?

38. What maternal and perinatal impacts are associated with pregnancy in women with systemic lupus erythematosus (SLE)?

39. What monitoring strategies would you implement for a woman with systemic lupus erythematosus (SLE) throughout pregnancy, childbirth, and the postpartum period?

40. What factors contribute to recurrent fetal loss?

41. Explain thrombophilia during pregnancy, including its definition and classification.

42. What is the therapeutic significance of low molecular weight heparin in managing recurrent pregnancy loss?

43. Explain the characteristics and significance of the Nitabuch's layer during pregnancy.

44. Discuss the diagnostic process for placenta accreta spectrum (PAS).

45. Detail the approach to managing placenta increta when diagnosed at 36 weeks of gestation.

46. List the possible causes or factors contributing to abruptio placentae.

47. Outline the management strategies for a patient diagnosed with placental abruption.
48. Define Placenta Accreta Syndrome (PAS) and discuss its clinical implications.
49. What factors increase the likelihood of developing Placenta Accreta Syndrome (PAS)?
50. What diagnostic methods would you employ to identify Placenta Accreta Syndrome (PAS)?
51. Strategies for managing Placenta Accreta Syndrome (PAS).
52. How is placenta accreta diagnosed using imaging techniques?
53. Approach to managing a patient with a history of previous cesarean section and suspected placenta accreta.
54. List the potential risk factors associated with placental abruption.
55. Could you explain the condition known as Couvelaire uterus?
56. Approach to treating placental abruption.
57. How would you manage a multigravida with a history of previous cesarean section, presenting with anterior type 3 placenta previa diagnosed at 28 weeks of gestation?
58. What antenatal care plan would you implement for this patient?
59. List the potential complications anticipated during cesarean section for this patient.
60. What management options are available if a morbidly adherent placenta is encountered during cesarean section for this patient?
61. How do you diagnose and treat a morbidly adherent placenta?
62. What are the different classifications of abnormal placental adhesion?
63. What diagnostic techniques are utilized and what treatment options are available for managing abnormal placental adhesion?
64. Key considerations in the surgical approach to managing placenta previa with accreta.
65. How can placenta previa be categorized?
66. What factors contribute to the development of placenta previa?

67. What methods would you utilize to verify the diagnosis of placenta previa?
68. What are the challenges associated with managing placenta previa?
69. What are the potential risk factors associated with placental abruption?
70. What diagnostic approaches would you use to identify placental abruption?
71. What potential adverse outcomes are associated with placental abruption?
72. What is the recommended management approach for a gravida 3, para 2, with 2 living children, admitted at 38 weeks of gestation with a diagnosis of placental abruption?
73. Please provide a definition and classification of morbidly adherent placenta (MAP).
74. How do ultrasound and MRI contribute to diagnosing morbidly adherent placenta (MAP)?
75. What potential adverse outcomes are associated with morbidly adherent placenta (MAP), and what strategies would you employ to manage them?
76. Explain the pathophysiological mechanisms underlying pre-eclampsia during pregnancy and its classification.
77. Provide a definition of preeclampsia?
78. Discuss the systemic complications associated with preeclampsia, considering its underlying pathophysiology.
79. Outline the management approach for a primigravida at 34 weeks of gestation presenting with eclampsia.
80. Categorize and provide definitions for hypertensive disorders occurring during pregnancy?
81. What is the role of antihypertensive medications in the management of preeclampsia?
82. Explain the underlying mechanisms involved in the development of pre-eclampsia?
83. What are the potential adverse outcomes associated with pre-eclampsia, and what measures can be taken to prevent them?

84. Differential diagnosis and management approach for HELLP syndrome.
85. List the potential causes of seizures occurring during pregnancy.
86. What are the potential maternal and fetal complications associated with eclampsia?
87. Outline the management plan for a primigravida at 32 weeks of gestation who is admitted with eclampsia.
88. A pregnant woman at 7 months gestation presents with a blood pressure reading of 140/100 mmHg.
89. List the potential reasons for generalized edema in a primigravida at full term of pregnancy.
90. Outline the clinical characteristics associated with severe preeclampsia?
91. What preventive measures can be taken to reduce the risk of eclampsia in pregnant women diagnosed with severe preeclampsia?
92. Describe the development or origin of twin-twin transfusion syndrome (TTTS)?
93. What diagnostic methods are used to identify cases of twin-twin transfusion syndrome (TTTS)?
94. Outline the approach to managing twin-twin transfusion syndrome (TTTS) in a primigravida with a twin pregnancy at 24 weeks of gestation.
95. Elaborate on the development or origin of twin pregnancies?
96. What potential adverse outcomes are associated with monochorionic twin pregnancies?
97. Describe the staging system developed by Quintero for twin-to-twin transfusion syndrome (TTTS)?
98. Current approaches to managing twin-to-twin transfusion syndrome (TTTS).
99. What techniques are utilized to determine chorionicity in pregnancies?
100. How does chorionicity affect the management approach for twin pregnancies?

101. Enumerate the various prenatal complications associated with twin pregnancies.
102. Postpartum assessment and management following the delivery of the first baby?
103. Approach to managing a pregnancy with triplets?
104. A 38-year-old patient presents to you with a triplet pregnancy at 6 weeks gestation, which was conceived through in vitro fertilization.
105. What key counseling points would you provide regarding antenatal care management in the first trimester and screening for aneuploidy in this scenario of a 38-year-old patient with a triplet pregnancy conceived through in vitro fertilization?
106. Enumerate the potential adverse outcomes associated with multiple pregnancies.
107. What antenatal monitoring strategies would you employ to assess the well-being of both the mother and fetuses in a multiple pregnancy?
108. List the potential risks to the fetus(es) in a twin pregnancy.
109. What methods would you use and at what stage of pregnancy would you determine the chorionicity of a twin pregnancy?
110. What diagnostic approaches and management strategies would you employ for twin-to-twin transfusion syndrome (TTTS)?
111. List the potential complications and discuss the management options for a monochorionic twin pregnancy.
112. List the factors that contribute to the higher occurrence of twin pregnancies.
113. What methods would you use to establish the chorionicity and amnionicity of a multiple pregnancy?
114. Provide an overview of TTTS (Twin-to-Twin Transfusion Syndrome) and its stages?
115. What are the approaches to managing TTTS (Twin-to-Twin Transfusion Syndrome) and what is the prognosis associated with it?
116. Approach to managing twins who exhibit discordance in growth or development.

117. Explain the concept of multifetal pregnancy reduction?

118. What is the objective of multifetal pregnancy reduction, and what are the technique and precautions involved in the procedure?

119. Describe the condition known as twin reversed arterial perfusion (TRAP sequence).

120. Explain the concepts of zygosity and chorionicity in the context of twin pregnancies?

121. Outline the management approach for a case involving a monoamniotic, monochorionic twin pregnancy.

122. What alterations occur in carbohydrate metabolism throughout pregnancy?

123. What is gestational diabetes mellitus (GDM)?

124. What are the recommended strategies for the management of diabetes mellitus diagnosed during pregnancy?

125. Explain the various approaches to screening for gestational diabetes mellitus.

126. Outline the potential adverse outcomes in neonates born to mothers with diabetes.

127. A 34-year-old woman with Type 2 Diabetes mellitus, currently managed with oral hypoglycemic agents (OHA), presents for her first antenatal care (ANC) visit at 6 weeks gestation.

128. What does current research indicate about the efficacy and safety of oral hypoglycemic agents (OHA) during pregnancy?

129. Detail the antenatal surveillance protocol for monitoring hyperglycemia and devise a management strategy for this woman.

130. Discuss the various approaches utilized to screen for gestational diabetes mellitus during pregnancy.

131. What are the potential adverse effects of elevated blood sugar levels on both maternal health and fetal development during pregnancy?

132. Discuss the comprehensive management approach for diabetes mellitus during pregnancy.

133. Explain the strategies for addressing shoulder dystocia in a fetus with macrosomia.

134. Describe the recommended screening procedures for gestational diabetes mellitus (GDM).
135. Discuss the utilization of medications for managing gestational diabetes mellitus (GDM).
136. Approaches to treating diabetic ketoacidosis.
137. Explain the alterations in carbohydrate metabolism observed in Gestational Diabetes Mellitus (GDM).
138. Outline the screening methods for gestational diabetes mellitus (GDM) in both high-risk and low-risk pregnant women.
139. List the measures necessary to attain optimal blood sugar management in gestational diabetes mellitus (GDM).
140. Describe the prenatal care considerations for a 33-year-old primigravida with a BMI of 38 kg/m^2 presenting at 6 weeks of pregnancy, with no significant medical history.
141. Anticipated antenatal and intrapartum challenges for the described case.
142. Discuss the perioperative care plan for a cesarean section in the described patient.
143. Outline pre-conception counseling considerations for a 31-year-old morbidly obese patient planning to undergo bariatric surgery.
144. What advice and guidance would you provide to the patient during pre-conception counseling before bariatric surgery?
145. What are the potential pregnancy-related challenges in a patient who has undergone bariatric surgery?
146. What dietary guidance would you offer to a young, low-risk primigravida during pregnancy?
147. What are the impacts of obesity on the course of pregnancy?
148. Guidelines for managing obstetric care in a pregnant patient with a history of previous bariatric surgery.
149. What factors contribute to the increased risk of blood clot formation during pregnancy?
150. Enumerate the factors that increase the likelihood of venous thromboembolism during pregnancy and the postpartum period.

151. Outline the strategies for preventing blood clot formation during pregnancy.

152. Explain why pregnancy is associated with an increased risk of blood clot formation.

153. Describe the importance of thromboprophylaxis for postpartum patients.

154. Identify the factors that contribute to the risk of venous thromboembolism in obstetrics and gynecology.

155. How can I effectively manage venous thromboembolism (VTE) risk in clinical practice?

156. What are the key clinical indicators for suspecting pulmonary thromboembolism, and what steps should be taken for its management?

157. What are the recommended strategies for preventing thrombotic complications in pregnant individuals?

158. What are the factors that increase the risk of thromboembolism during pregnancy and the postpartum period?

159. What are the recommended management strategies for a pregnant individual who is gravida 2, para 1, with a history of deep vein thrombosis (DVT) during a previous pregnancy?

160. What are the diagnostic approaches used to identify deep vein thrombosis (DVT) in pregnant individuals?

161. Describe the management protocol for deep vein thrombosis (DVT) in a first-time pregnant individual at 30 weeks gestation.

162. What criteria does the World Health Organization (WHO) use to classify the risk of heart diseases during pregnancy?

163. Detail the approach to managing a 23-year-old first-time pregnant individual at 20 weeks gestation diagnosed with rheumatic heart disease and mitral stenosis, who underwent mechanical valve replacement three years ago and currently presents with NYHA class 3 functional status.

164. What does preconception counseling involve?

165. What are the key considerations for providing preconception counseling to a 24-year-old woman who is nulliparous and has rheumatic heart disease with mitral stenosis?

166. What are the signs and symptoms that may suggest the presence of heart disease during pregnancy?

167. What are the recommended management approaches for severe mitral stenosis diagnosed during the second trimester of pregnancy?

168. What changes occur in the cardiovascular system during pregnancy?

169. What diagnostic methods are utilized to identify cardiac conditions during pregnancy?

170. Outline the approach to managing pregnant individuals with a prosthetic mitral valve.

171. What are the diagnostic criteria and recommended strategies for managing peripartum cardiomyopathy?

172. What effects does mitral stenosis have on pregnant women?

173. What factors might prompt corrective intervention for this condition during pregnancy?

174. What post-procedural care would you provide for a patient who underwent mitral valvuloplasty during the fifth month of pregnancy?

175. What are the different classifications of heart diseases based on functional status?

176. What are the considerations for managing labor in women diagnosed with rheumatic heart disease?

177. What is the significance of anticoagulant therapy for pregnant patients with prosthetic heart valves?

178. What are the alterations in hemodynamics that occur during pregnancy?

179. How does mitral stenosis impact pregnancy outcomes and maternal health?

180. What preventive strategies can be implemented to mitigate risks and complications in pregnant women diagnosed with mitral stenosis?

181. When should anticoagulant therapy be initiated, and which agents are recommended for pregnant women with prosthetic heart valves, and what are the reasons for their use?

182. What monitoring protocols would you implement for a 20-year-old primigravida at 14 weeks gestation with rheumatic heart disease

and mitral stenosis, throughout her pregnancy, delivery, and postpartum period?

183. What are the signs and symptoms that may suggest the presence of heart disease in pregnant individuals?

184. What is the New York Heart Association (NYHA) classification system used for heart disease, and how does it relate to prognosis?

185. What contraceptive recommendations would you provide to a woman with mitral stenosis who is being discharged after delivery?

186. What factors contribute to early neonatal mortality in preterm infants?

187. Detail the management approach for a 31-year-old woman, gravida 3, para 2, with a history of preterm early neonatal deaths in previous pregnancies, presenting to the antenatal care outpatient department at 25 weeks of gestation.

188. How is premature rupture of membranes diagnosed?

189. Outline the management protocol for a first-time pregnant individual at 30 weeks gestation who presents with suspected amniotic fluid leakage.

190. What factors contribute to the likelihood of preterm birth?

191. Discuss the adverse outcomes associated with preterm birth.

192. What strategies can be implemented to reduce the complications associated with preterm birth?

193. What are the clinical signs and symptoms suggestive of preterm labor?

194. Strategies for anticipating and averting preterm labor?

195. What is the function and use of Atosiban in obstetrics?

196. What does the term PPROM stand for?

197. What factors contribute to preterm premature rupture of membranes (PPROM)?

198. What diagnostic methods are employed to verify the occurrence of preterm premature rupture of membranes (PPROM)?

199. What is the recommended management approach for a patient diagnosed with preterm premature rupture of membranes (PPROM) at 33 weeks of gestation?

200. What are the primary short-term and long-term challenges associated with infants born with very low birth weight?
201. What are the underlying mechanisms involved in the onset of preterm labor?
202. What approaches can be taken to reduce the risk of preterm birth?
203. What factors contribute to the occurrence of preterm premature rupture of membranes (PPROM)?
204. What steps would you take in the management of a patient diagnosed with preterm premature rupture of membranes (PPROM) at 28 weeks of pregnancy?
205. What is cervical insufficiency and its causes?
206. What diagnostic methods and management strategies would you employ for a patient presenting with cervical insufficiency at 14 weeks of pregnancy?
207. What are the key aspects of postoperative care following a cerclage procedure?
208. What is abdominal cerclage surgery?
209. A first-time pregnant woman at 8 months of gestation presents with vaginal leakage.
210. What diagnostic steps would you take to ascertain the cause of vaginal leakage in a primigravida at 8 months of gestation?
211. What tests or examinations would you consider in evaluating the cause of vaginal leakage in a primigravida at 8 months of gestation?
212. What management approach would you take for the patient experiencing vaginal leakage at 8 months of pregnancy?
213. What methods can be utilized to identify pregnant women who may be at risk for spontaneous preterm labor?
214. What factors contribute to preterm labor, and what clinical signs indicate its occurrence?
215. What strategies can be implemented to reduce the risk of preterm labor?
216. What are the different types of medications utilized to inhibit preterm labor?

217. A primigravida patient who is not registered for prenatal care presents at 32 weeks of pregnancy with an intrauterine device (IUD).
218. What factors might lead to the presence of an intrauterine device (IUD) in this patient at 32 weeks of pregnancy?
219. What potential issues or adverse outcomes may arise from the presence of an intrauterine device (IUD) in this patient?
220. What steps would you take to address the situation with this patient?
221. What factors contribute to stillbirth?
222. What methods can be used to assess a stillborn infant?
223. What counseling would you provide to the parents in this situation?
224. What factors contribute to the occurrence of stillbirths?
225. What assessments would you conduct for a patient with a history of previous stillbirths?
226. What are the factors that can lead to fetal hydrops?
227. Outline the diagnostic process and treatment approach for immune fetal hydrops in a patient at 22 weeks' gestation.
228. What is the definition of Rh isoimmunization in pregnancy?
229. Describe the available management strategies for a pregnant woman who is Gravid 2, Para 1, and Rh isoimmunized at 30 weeks of gestation.
230. Outline the approach to managing a neonate with Rh isoimmunization.
231. What factors contribute to feto-maternal hemorrhage?
232. What methods are used to assess feto-maternal hemorrhage?
233. Can you explain the utilization of Routine Antenatal Anti-D Prophylaxis (RAADP), including dosage considerations?
234. What are the factors involved in the etiology and pathogenesis of non-immune hydrops?
235. What steps would you take in the management of a patient diagnosed with non-immune hydrops at 26 weeks of pregnancy?
236. What is feto-maternal hemorrhage, and how does it impact a woman who is Rh negative?

237. What are the factors contributing to feto-maternal hemorrhage?
238. What is the method for determining the appropriate dosage of anti-D to prevent Rh isoimmunization?
239. What are the non-invasive and invasive methods used to detect fetal isoimmunization in pregnancies involving Rh-negative individuals?
240. What is the purpose of intrauterine fetal blood transfusion?
241. What do you understand by Rh incompatibility?
242. Detail the management approach for Rh incompatibility during the antenatal period and labor & delivery in a primigravida woman who is Rh negative.
243. What factors contribute to the development of hydrops fetalis, and what is its underlying physiological mechanism?
244. What steps would you take in the management of a pregnant woman who is Rh negative and has been diagnosed with hydrops fetalis at 32 weeks of gestation?
245. What is Small for Gestational Age (SGA) and what causes it?
246. How should a pregnant woman with suspected fetal growth restriction at 28 weeks of gestation be evaluated and managed?
247. What is fetal growth restriction and its causes?
248. What is the management approach for fetal growth restriction diagnosed at 32 weeks of gestation?
249. What are the complications associated with a small for gestational age (SGA) fetus?
250. What are the different methods used to evaluate the risks associated with a small for gestational age (SGA) fetus?
251. What are the evidence-based guidelines for managing a case of a small for gestational age (SGA) fetus?
252. What does IUGR mean in the context of pregnancy?
253. What are the methods for fetal surveillance during the antenatal period?
254. What is intrauterine growth restriction?
255. How are Doppler flow studies used in managing intrauterine growth restriction (IUGR)?

256. What are the perinatal complications associated with intrauterine growth restriction (IUGR) babies?

257. What is the role of ferric carboxymaltose in treating anemia during pregnancy and the postpartum period?

258. How can different types of microcytic anemia be differentiated in pregnant women, and what are the treatments for each type?

259. What are the complications associated with anemia in pregnancy?

260. How would you investigate and manage a case of a multigravida with a hemoglobin level of 6 g% at 30 weeks of pregnancy who has not received any antenatal care?

261. What are the maternal and fetal complications associated with severe anemia (Hb 3g%) in a primigravida at 36 weeks of gestation?

262. How should a primigravida with severe anemia at 36 weeks of gestation be investigated and managed?

263. What does thalassemia refer to?

264. What are the recommended methods for screening for thalassemia during pregnancy?

265. How should pregnant women with thalassemia trait be managed?

266. How should a pregnancy be investigated and managed if both parents are carriers of thalassemia?

267. What is the approach for investigating and managing severe anemia in a pregnant woman at 32 weeks of gestation?

268. What is thrombocytopenia in the context of pregnancy?

269. How is thrombocytopenia classified etiologically in pregnancy?

270. What are the diagnostic and management considerations for gestational thrombocytopenia?

271. What causes thrombocytopenia during pregnancy?

272. How should a case of thrombocytopenia in pregnancy be evaluated?

273. How is immune thrombocytopenic purpura (ITP) managed during pregnancy?

274. What are the physiological skin changes that occur during pregnancy?

275. What are the causes of pruritus in pregnancy?

276. What is the pathophysiology and management of intrahepatic cholestasis of pregnancy (IHCP)?

277. How is post-partum thyroiditis diagnosed and managed?

278. How is hypothyroidism managed during pregnancy?

279. What are the physiological changes in thyroid function during pregnancy?

280. What complications can arise for both the mother and fetus due to hypothyroidism during pregnancy?

281. How should overt hypothyroidism in pregnant women be managed?

282. What are the underlying causes and mechanisms of pyelonephritis during pregnancy?

283. Explore the diagnostic methods, treatment strategies, and potential complications associated with pyelonephritis during pregnancy.

284. Examine the alterations in renal physiology that occur during pregnancy.

285. Explain the mechanisms involved in the development of Acute Kidney Injury (AKI).

286. What is the clinical significance of asymptomatic bacteriuria?

287. How should acute renal failure be addressed in pregnant individuals?

288. Explore the diagnostic process, potential complications, and recommended management strategies for acute pyelonephritis in pregnant individuals.

289. What alterations occur in the urinary tract during pregnancy as a result of physiological changes?

290. Describe asymptomatic bacteriuria and its implications for pregnant individuals.

291. What are the recommended approaches for the management of acute pyelonephritis during pregnancy?

292. Outline the potential maternal and fetal complications that may arise during pregnancy in a woman who has undergone renal transplantation.

293. What are the recommended methods for monitoring a pregnancy in a woman who has undergone renal transplantation?

294. Develop a comprehensive plan for the delivery of a woman who has undergone renal transplantation.
295. Describe the alterations observed in the urinary system, both anatomically and physiologically, throughout pregnancy.
296. Explain the clinical significance and implications of asymptomatic bacteriuria.
297. What impact does asymptomatic bacteriuria have on pregnancy outcomes?
298. Detail the recommended approach for managing asymptomatic bacteriuria.
299. Discuss the alterations in renal function that occur as part of the physiological changes during a typical pregnancy.
300. List the factors contributing to the development of acute renal failure (ARF) in pregnant individuals.
301. Detail the recommended strategies for addressing acute renal failure (ARF) in pregnant women.
302. Explain the clinical presentation and significance of hyperemesis gravidarum during pregnancy.
303. What are the characteristic symptoms and potential adverse outcomes associated with hyperemesis gravidarum?
304. Describe the recommended approaches for managing hyperemesis gravidarum during pregnancy.
305. Examine the conditions that may present similarly to hyperemesis gravidarum and discuss their differential diagnosis.
306. List the factors contributing to dyspnea during pregnancy.
307. Discuss the reciprocal impact of bronchial asthma on pregnancy outcomes and the effects of pregnancy on the course of asthma.
308. What are the recommended management strategies for asthma during the process of labor?
309. Describe the progression and implications of epilepsy during pregnancy.
310. Examine the pharmacological agents commonly employed for managing epilepsy during pregnancy.
311. List the potential etiologies of seizures occurring during pregnancy.

312. What are the effects of epilepsy on pregnancy outcomes and maternal health?
313. Describe the fundamental principles guiding the management of medical conditions during pregnancy.
314. How should a person with a known history of epilepsy approach pregnancy planning?
315. What advice and guidance would you provide to a woman with epilepsy who is considering pregnancy?
316. How does epilepsy impact the course and outcomes of pregnancy?
317. Discuss the impact of antiepileptic medications on pregnancy outcomes and fetal development.
318. Detail the suggested approach for managing a woman with epilepsy during labor.
319. Explain the concept of pre-conception care and its relevance in clinical practice.
320. What diagnostic and therapeutic strategies would you employ for a woman with a history of congenital heart disease in a previous pregnancy?
321. Describe the concept and significance of pre-conception counseling.
322. Describe the role of pre-conceptional counselling in obstetrics?
323. What advice and guidance would you provide to a newly married woman diagnosed with rheumatic heart disease and mitral stenosis?
324. Explain the different approaches to antenatal fetal screening.
325. Explore non-invasive methods utilized for prenatal detection of fetal abnormalities.
326. What methods would you use to determine the gestational age of a pregnancy?
327. What are the recommended approaches for managing a pregnant woman who has surpassed her expected due date?
328. Define antenatal care and its significance in pregnancy management.
329. What are the essential diagnostic resources necessary for antenatal care in a tertiary healthcare setting?

330. What advice and guidance would you provide to a low-risk pregnant woman during the early stages of antenatal care?

331. What are the essential components required for establishing an optimal antenatal clinic within your local context?

332. What strategies would you suggest implementing to reduce the rate of attrition in a healthcare system?

333. A pregnant individual who is positive for Hepatitis B surface antigen (HBsAg) is admitted to the obstetric ward at 36 weeks of gestation.

334. What preventive measures would you implement to minimize the risk of transmission to healthcare providers while caring for a patient who is positive for Hepatitis B surface antigen (HBsAg) admitted to the obstetric ward at 36 weeks of gestation?

335. What strategies would you employ to minimize the risk of perinatal transmission of Hepatitis B virus from a mother who is positive for Hepatitis B surface antigen (HBsAg) to her neonate?

336. What factors contribute to the classification of pregnancy as high risk for women who test positive for Hepatitis B surface antigen (HBsAg)?

337. What are the recommended approaches for managing a woman who is positive for Hepatitis B surface antigen (HBsAg) during labor and delivery?

338. How should you approach the management of a newborn born to a mother who is positive for Hepatitis B surface antigen (HBsAg)?

339. What is maternal sepsis, and how would you diagnose and manage a 28-year-old woman who presents with severe sepsis 24 hours after a vaginal delivery that occurred at home in a village, attended by a traditional birth attendant (Dai)?:

340. Identify the factors that increase the risk of maternal sepsis.

341. Outline the diagnostic process and recommended management strategies for a suspected case of maternal sepsis.

342. What is the definition of postpartum fever? List the potential factors leading to postpartum fever.

343. What are the recommended management approaches for treating postpartum sepsis in a woman who has given birth for the first time?

344. Explain the concept of postpartum sepsis.

345. What are the factors that increase the likelihood of developing postpartum sepsis?

346. What are the recommended strategies for treating postpartum sepsis?

347. Define postpartum blues and its characteristics.

348. Identify the factors that increase the risk of postpartum depression and discuss its effects.

349. What are the recommended methods for managing postpartum depression?

350. What factors contribute to the development of postpartum sepsis?

351. What diagnostic steps would you take and what treatment approaches would you consider for a case suspected of postpartum sepsis?

352. Explain the potential long-term effects of postpartum sepsis on reproductive health.

353. Explain the underlying mechanisms involved in disseminated intravascular coagulation (DIC)?

354. What are the recommended approaches for treating disseminated intravascular coagulation (DIC)?

355. List the potential reasons for fever occurring during pregnancy and the postpartum period (puerperium).

356. What are the recommended strategies for managing malaria during pregnancy?

357. What are the common symptoms experienced by pregnant individuals with COVID-19 infection?

358. What are the considerations and recommendations regarding COVID-19 vaccination for pregnant individuals?

359. How should genital warts be managed in pregnant individuals?

360. What are the characteristics and implications of congenital rubella syndrome?

361. How are rubella infections diagnosed in pregnant women and in the fetus?

362. What steps would you take to manage a pregnant woman who has been exposed to rubella infection at 11 weeks of gestation?

363. How would you approach the management of pregnancy in a woman who contracted chickenpox at 26 weeks of gestation?

364. Examine the impact of malaria infection during pregnancy.

365. What are the potential complications of pregnancy that necessitate heightened monitoring?

366. What are the recommended approaches for treating malaria during pregnancy?

367. Explain the categorization of gestational trophoblastic diseases and the underlying mechanisms involved in their pathogenesis.

368. How would you approach the management of a patient diagnosed with a partial hydatidiform mole alongside a live fetus at 14 weeks of gestation?

369. Explain the causes and diagnostic methods for incompetent cervix, as well as the various types of cerclage procedures.

370. How would you manage cervical incompetence at 18 weeks of gestation in a patient with a history of recurrent pregnancy loss (RPL)?

371. Discuss the significance of the Umbilical Coiling Index in obstetrics.

372. Explain the different types of umbilical cord insertions in pregnancy.

373. Outline the diagnostic process and recommended treatment strategies for vasa previa.

374. What are the diagnostic methods used to identify a cesarean scar pregnancy?

375. What are the potential factors that increase the risk of developing a cesarean scar pregnancy?

376. Discuss the available approaches for managing cesarean scar pregnancies.

377. Can you explain the concept of non-immune hydrops fetalis (NIHF)?

378. What are the recommended management strategies for a case of non-immune hydrops fetalis (NIHF) diagnosed at 26 weeks of gestation, and at what gestational age would you consider delivery?

379. What factors contribute to decreased fetal movements during the third trimester of pregnancy?
380. How would you approach the management of decreased fetal movements in a first-time pregnant woman at 36 weeks of gestation?
381. What are the techniques used to determine the gestational age of a pregnancy?
382. What are the markers used to assess fetal maturity?
383. Explain the concept of a pregnancy of unknown location (PUL)?
384. Examine the effectiveness and implications of laparoscopic myomectomy in the treatment of uterine fibroids.
385. What are the factors that can lead to the formation of a weak surgical scar?
386. What approaches would you take in managing a pregnancy for a woman who has undergone laparoscopic myomectomy?
387. Provide a summary of the concept of exclusive breastfeeding?
388. Provide a summary of postpartum thyroid disorders?
389. Provide a summary of strategies to prevent Rh isoimmunization?

OBSTETRIC EMERGENCIES

1. Examine the factors contributing to maternal collapse during pregnancy.
2. Explore the strategies for managing maternal collapse.
3. Define maternal near-miss incidents and enumerate their diverse causes.
4. Outline the diagnostic protocol for sudden maternal collapse during labor.
5. Managing resuscitation in a critically ill patient with late-stage pregnancy.
6. Addressing abrupt postpartum collapse and its therapeutic approach.
7. Define postpartum collapse and elucidate its characteristics.

8. List the various factors contributing to postpartum collapse.
9. Detail the approach to managing amniotic fluid embolism in a primiparous woman immediately following delivery.
10. Describe the clinical management of a young multigravida presenting to the emergency department with sudden and severe shortness of breath during her full-term pregnancy.
11. Explore potential differential diagnoses for a young multigravida presenting with acute and severe breathlessness in the emergency department during her full-term pregnancy.
12. Outline the diagnostic evaluation process employed to determine the underlying cause of acute and severe breathlessness in the young multigravida presenting in the emergency department during her full-term pregnancy.
13. Discuss the pathogenesis of amniotic fluid embolism.
14. Describe the management strategies and long-term outcomes associated with amniotic fluid embolism.
15. Define postpartum collapse and elucidate its characteristics.
16. List the various factors contributing to postpartum collapse.
17. Detail the management approach for a primiparous woman experiencing amniotic fluid embolism immediately following delivery.
18. Define postpartum collapse and list its potential causes.
19. Discuss the management approach for amniotic fluid embolism in a primiparous woman immediately following delivery.
20. Explain the physiological mechanisms underlying the development of amniotic fluid embolism
21. List the various factors that contribute to the development of oligohydramnios.
22. Describe the management approach for a primigravida at 34 weeks of pregnancy with an amniotic fluid index (AFI) of 5 cm.
23. A woman who is pregnant for the second time and has given birth once, currently at 38 weeks of gestation, and has a previous history of cesarean section scar, presents with a complaint of decreased fetal movements.

24. Enumerate potential differential diagnoses for the described case of a woman at 38 weeks of gestation, gravida 2 para 1, with a previous cesarean section scar, presenting with decreased fetal movements.
25. Examine the diverse management options for the potential differential diagnoses in the presented case of a woman at 38 weeks of gestation, gravida 2 para 1, with a previous cesarean section scar, presenting with decreased fetal movements
26. Explain uterine rupture, including its diagnosis and management strategies.
27. Define Bandl's ring and elucidate its significance in obstetrics.
28. Discuss the clinical presentation and therapeutic strategies for uterine rupture.
29. List the various factors contributing to the retention of the placenta
30. Examine the diverse management strategies available for addressing retained placenta.
31. Outline the classification system used for uterine inversion.
32. Examine the therapeutic approaches for addressing uterine inversion that occurs subsequent to vaginal delivery.
33. Explore the clinical aspects and management of acute uterine inversion.
34. Strategies for addressing postpartum hemorrhage.
35. What is meant by acute uterine inversion?
36. Enumerate the risk factors, describe the diagnostic process, and delineate the management plan for acute uterine inversion.
37. What are the circumstances that may necessitate a peripartum hysterectomy?
38. Discuss the potential adverse outcomes linked with peripartum hysterectomy.
39. Describe the postoperative care plan following peripartum hysterectomy.
40. Enumerate the criteria necessitating peripartum hysterectomy.
41. Examine the implications of significant blood loss in obstetric situations.

42. What is meant by significant blood loss in obstetrics?
43. What methods can be utilized to assess blood loss accurately?
44. Discuss the importance of prompt management during the critical period following obstetric emergencies.
45. Outline the procedures involved in initiating resuscitative measures.
46. Enumerate the factors contributing to postpartum hemorrhage.
47. Detail the approach to managing a case of postpartum hemorrhage that does not respond to uterotonic medications.
48. List the potential adverse effects associated with blood transfusions.
49. Explore the role of bilateral ligation of internal iliac arteries in obstetric management.
50. Criteria for determining the eligibility of a patient for admission to an intensive care unit.
51. Enumerate the etiological factors contributing to significant obstetric hemorrhage.
52. Detail the emergency obstetric interventions for managing atonic postpartum hemorrhage.
53. Describe the immediate and delayed complications associated with atonic postpartum hemorrhage.
54. Enumerate the adverse outcomes associated with extensive blood transfusions.
55. Elucidate the concept of deep transverse arrest (DTA) and explore its diverse causes.
56. Examine the available strategies for managing deep transverse arrest (DTA).
57. Detail the potential complications that may arise in a neonate following delivery complicated by deep transverse arrest (DTA).
58. Define obstructive labor and list its contributing factors.
59. What diagnostic methods are utilized to identify obstructive labor?
60. List the maternal and fetal complications associated with obstructed labor.
61. What is obstetric shock?

62. List the etiological factors and stages of endotoxic shock.
63. Discuss the management approach for a pregnant patient presenting with septic shock.
64. List the etiological factors and outline the therapeutic interventions for managing septic shock in obstetrics.
65. What are some devices or methods used to manage shock in obstetrics?
66. Explain the application of these devices in obstetrics and gynecology.
67. Define peripartum cardiomyopathy.
68. Outline the clinical characteristics and long-term outlook associated with peripartum cardiomyopathy.
69. Discuss the therapeutic approach for managing congestive heart failure in the context of peripartum cardiomyopathy during full-term pregnancy.

Chapter - 2

GYNECOLOGY

PREGNANCY

1. What leads to repeated miscarriages?
2. What is the importance of a pedigree chart?
3. What role does genetic counseling play in addressing recurrent pregnancy loss?
4. What would be the medical approach for a 31-year-old woman experiencing two miscarriages and difficulties conceiving?
5. What are the potential reasons for recurrent pregnancy loss and how are they assessed?
6. What are the treatment options for a blocked fallopian tube?
7. How is persistent vulvovaginal candidiasis treated?
8. What are the natural defense mechanisms of the genital tract?
9. What leads to itching of the vulva?
10. How is moniliasis diagnosed and treated?
11. What is the difference between physiological and pathological vaginal discharge?
12. How is vaginal discharge diagnosed to accurately determine the cause in a woman of reproductive age?
13. What are the treatments for different types of vaginal discharge?
14. How does the normal vaginal ecosystem function?
15. What are the potential health impacts of disruptions in the normal vaginal ecosystem?
16. What are the diagnostic and management strategies for bacterial vaginosis?
17. What constitutes normal vaginal discharge in a young woman?

18. How does the female genital tract protect against ascending infections?
19. How is vulvo-vaginal candidiasis treated?
20. What are the typical microorganisms found in the normal vaginal flora?
21. What factors increase the risk of vulvo-vaginal candidiasis, and what methods are used for its diagnosis?
22. What steps should be taken to evaluate and manage a woman experiencing recurrent vulvo-vaginal candidiasis?
23. How is recurrent vulvo-vaginal candidiasis treated?
24. What are the potential differential diagnoses and management strategies for a 25-year-old female, P1L1, experiencing acute lower abdominal pain with a history of irregular periods, chronic pelvic pain post-LSCS, and treatment for Koch's disease?
25. What are the causes and treatment options for chronic pelvic pain in reproductive-aged women?
26. What is the difference between ovarian remnant syndrome and residual ovary syndrome?
27. Management of a 29-year-old woman with chronic pelvic pain, dyspareunia, and painful menstruation?
28. How should chronic pelvic pain be managed?
29. What could contribute to the development of chronic pelvic pain?
30. What approach would you take to assess and treat chronic pelvic pain in a 26-year-old woman experiencing secondary infertility?
31. What approach would you take to treat acute pelvic pain in a 22-year-old woman?
32. What are the potential complications and long-term effects of acute pelvic inflammatory disease (PID) in women?
33. What do the CDC guidelines state regarding the diagnosis of acute PID and the criteria for hospital admission?
34. How does contraceptive use affect the risk of developing pelvic inflammatory disease (PID)?
35. What are the causes of pelvic inflammatory disease (PID) in young women of reproductive age?

36. What are symptoms, signs and management of PID?
37. What are the long-term consequences of pelvic inflammatory disease (PID) and how can they be prevented?
38. What criteria does the CDC use for the diagnosis of pelvic inflammatory disease (PID)?
39. What criteria indicate hospital admission for pelvic inflammatory disease (PID)?
40. What microbes commonly cause acute salpingitis?
41. Understanding and Grading Acute Salpingitis through Laparoscopy: What's the Process?
42. How does delaying treatment increase the risk of infertility?
43. What is Pelvic Inflammatory Disease (PID) and its implications?
44. What approaches are used for diagnosing and treating Pelvic Inflammatory Disease (PID)?
45. What causes acute Pelvic Inflammatory Disease (PID)?
46. What are the symptoms of Pelvic Inflammatory Disease (PID) and how is it differentiated from other conditions?
47. How is Pelvic Inflammatory Disease (PID) treated and what are its potential long-term effects?
48. What does the PALM-COEIN classification system detail regarding abnormal uterine bleeding?
49. What are the non-surgical treatment options for uterine fibroids?
50. A 31-year-old patient experiences abnormal uterine bleeding, and biopsy shows endometrial hyperplasia with atypia. She wishes to maintain fertility. How should her condition be managed?
51. What are the risk factors for developing endometrial hyperplasia?
52. What treatment options are available for a patient with endometrial hyperplasia?
53. What should be the follow-up care protocol for a patient with endometrial hyperplasia?
54. What leads to excessive menstrual bleeding?
55. How would you assess a case of abnormal heavy menstrual bleeding in a 33-year-old woman with multiple childbirths?

56. What are the treatment options available for managing heavy menstrual bleeding (HMB)?
57. What are the various classifications of endometrial hyperplasia?
58. What are the management strategies for different types of endometrial hyperplasia in a peri-menopausal woman?
59. What does the FIGO classification system (PALM-COEIN) represent for identifying causes of abnormal uterine bleeding in non-pregnant women of reproductive age?
60. How is AUB-A managed in a 37-year-old woman experiencing severe heavy menstrual bleeding?
61. What mechanisms control menstrual blood loss at the endometrial level?
62. What non-surgical treatment options are available for managing uterine fibroids?
63. What are the potential causes of menometrorrhagia in a 44-year-old woman with multiple pregnancies?
64. What investigations would you conduct for a 44-year-old multiparous woman with menometrorrhagia?
65. What is the approach to managing a submucosal fibroid polyp?
66. A woman presents with heavy menstrual bleeding and infertility; examination shows a large myoma at the uterine fundus. How would you proceed?
67. What is the rationale for choosing surgical management in this case of heavy menstrual bleeding and infertility with a large myoma at the uterine fundus?
68. What are the preoperative preparations and potential complications associated with the surgical removal of a uterine myoma?
69. What is the classification and management approach for a case of uterine fibroids?
70. What are the different non-invasive treatment options for Leiomyoma?
71. What are the possible causes of anuria following an abdominal hysterectomy in a 46-year-old woman with a history of cervical fibroid?

72. What could lead to the absence of urine production?
73. What are the key approaches to managing anuria?
74. What potential complications might arise in a 46-year-old woman following an abdominal hysterectomy for a cervical fibroid, particularly in the context of postoperative anuria?
75. How can blood loss be reduced during a myomectomy?
76. What does the term leiomyomatosis refer to?
77. What is the function of power morcellation in the treatment of uterine fibroids?
78. What is the latest classification system for Abnormal Uterine Bleeding (AUB)?
79. How is fibromyoma typically managed?
80. What are the different classifications of cervical fibroids?
81. What potential complications can arise during surgery for a cervical fibroid, and what preventive measures can be taken?
82. What approaches can be employed to reduce blood loss during a myomectomy procedure?
83. What factors make a myomectomy the preferred choice for women of reproductive age?
84. What is the current standing of uterine artery embolization as a treatment for fibroids?
85. What are the different stages of endometriosis?
86. What are the non-invasive methods for diagnosing endometriosis?
87. What are the treatment options for a 32-year-old patient after undergoing definitive surgery for endometriosis?
88. What causes endometriosis, and what are its symptoms?
89. What conditions would necessitate surgical intervention for endometriosis?
90. Explain the surgical approaches used in treating endometriosis?
91. What are the challenges and precautions associated with performing a laparoscopic cystectomy on an infertile woman with large endometriomas on both ovaries?

92. What are the theories behind the development of endometriosis?

93. What is the role of genetics in the development of endometriosis?

94. What are the medical treatment options for endometriosis?

95. How does laparoscopy contribute to the management of endometriosis?

96. What steps are involved in evaluating fertility in a woman with endometriosis?

97. What causes endometriosis and how is it diagnosed?

98. What are the non-surgical treatment options for endometriosis?

99. What causes endometriosis and how is laparoscopy used in its diagnosis?

100. What are the medical treatment options for ectopic pregnancy?

101. What is a cesarean scar pregnancy?

102. What are the latest developments in treating tubal ectopic pregnancy?

103. What are the different treatment options for ectopic pregnancy?

104. What are the different surgical approaches used in the treatment of ectopic pregnancy?

105. What are the various classifications of ectopic pregnancy?

106. How would you evaluate a patient with a suspected ectopic pregnancy in an emergency setting?

107. How is an early unruptured tubal ectopic pregnancy diagnosed and treated?

108. How is an unruptured tubal ectopic pregnancy diagnosed?

109. What are the approaches to managing an unruptured tubal ectopic pregnancy without immediate intervention?

110. What are the implications of continued trophoblastic activity after treating an ectopic pregnancy?

111. What is an ectopic pregnancy, and what are the different types of ectopic pregnancies?

112. What factors contribute to the rising incidence of unruptured ectopic pregnancies?

113. What are the recommended management strategies for a nulliparous patient?
114. What are the applications of laser technology in gynecology?
115. What diagnostic procedures are typically employed in cases where genital tuberculosis is suspected?
116. What are the symptoms and signs associated with pelvic tuberculosis?
117. What diagnostic methods are typically used to identify pelvic tuberculosis?
118. What are the approaches to managing pelvic tuberculosis?
119. What are the typical clinical manifestations of genital tuberculosis in young women of reproductive age?
120. What are the latest developments in laboratory techniques for diagnosing genital tuberculosis?
121. What are the reasons prompting surgical intervention in women with genital tuberculosis?
122. Discuss the effectiveness of different Nuclear Amplification Assays (NAA) for diagnosing endometrial tuberculosis.
123. Explain what multi-drug resistant tuberculosis (MDR-TB) and extensively drug-resistant tuberculosis (XDR-TB) are, and discuss the challenges involved in managing these cases.
124. What treatment options are available for infertility caused by genital tuberculosis, and what are their respective success rates?
125. Describe the typical microbial composition found in the vagina.
126. Managing recurrent vulvovaginal candidiasis.
127. What are the reasons for ulcers on the vulva?
128. What steps would you take in the clinical evaluation of a case with vulval ulcers, and how would you confirm your diagnosis?
129. What are the strategies for managing vulval ulcers?
130. What are the various categories of ulcers found in the genital area?
131. How does the clinical presentation of genital ulcers vary with different diagnoses?

132. What are the varieties of genital ulcers that are transmitted through sexual contact?

133. What are the clinical characteristics of each type of sexually transmitted genital ulcer?

134. What methods are used to definitively diagnose sexually transmitted genital ulcers?

135. What is pyometra?

136. How is pyometra diagnosed and managed?

137. What leads to the development of pyometra?

138. What are the possible diagnoses and management strategies for a 35-year-old female patient presenting with prolapse and irregular bleeding 8 months post-normal vaginal delivery?

139. How is vulvodynia defined?

140. What are the different classifications of vulvodynia?

141. What are the treatment strategies for localized vulvodynia?

142. What are the reasons for itching associated with vulvodynia?

143. What is the approach to managing a patient with a white patch on the labia minora?

144. How does colposcopy contribute to the management of vulvar lesions?

145. What are the benefits and risks of prophylactic salpingectomy?

146. What are the reasons behind bleeding after sexual intercourse?

147. What are the steps for investigating and managing post-coital bleeding in a 45-year-old woman?

148. What are the key parameters a gynecologist should evaluate during a health check-up of a 61-year-old woman, and why are these important?

149. What guidance should be provided to a 61-year-old woman following a health check-up with normal findings?

UROGYNECOLOGY

1. What is stress urinary incontinence (SUI)?
2. Explain the causes and methods for assessing stress urinary incontinence (SUI)?
3. Provide an analysis of the vaginal surgical procedures utilized in treating stress urinary incontinence (SUI)?
4. Explain the drug treatments used for overactive bladder?
5. How does bladder continence work?
6. What is stress urinary incontinence, and how is it caused and assessed?
7. How would you approach the treatment of stress urinary incontinence in a 41-year-old woman who has never given birth?
8. How does urinary continence function in females?
9. How is urinary retention treated in the first trimester of pregnancy?
10. Explain what extramural incontinence is?
11. What leads to the formation of a vesicovaginal fistula?
12. How is a vesicovaginal fistula assessed and treated?
13. Explain the range of conditions and underlying causes associated with pelvic floor dysfunction.
14. Explain the underlying mechanisms, how to diagnose, and treat disorders related to an overly tight pelvic floor.
15. What is involved in a urodynamic study?
16. How is genuine stress urinary incontinence treated?
17. Explain the underlying mechanisms that lead to urinary incontinence?
18. What are the drug treatments for managing an overactive bladder?
19. What leads to stress urinary incontinence in middle-aged individuals?
20. What methods are used to diagnose stress urinary incontinence?
21. What are the modern approaches to treating stress urinary incontinence?
22. What medications are used to treat an overactive bladder?
23. How is biofeedback therapy used in treating pelvic floor dysfunction?

24. How does physiotherapy benefit women after childbirth?
25. How does urinary incontinence occur from a physiological perspective?
26. What steps would you take to assess incontinence in a 54-year-old woman who has given birth?
27. What treatment options are available for stress incontinence in a middle-aged woman who has had children?
28. Explain how the process of urination works?
29. What causes an overactive bladder from an etiological and pathogenetic perspective?
30. What are the methods for diagnosing and managing an overactive bladder?
31. Explain what stress incontinence is?
32. Explain the causes and assessment methods for stress incontinence?
33. What is the strategy for treating stress incontinence?
34. How does urinary incontinence occur from a physiological standpoint?
35. What steps would you take to assess urge incontinence in a 54-year-old woman who has given birth?
36. How is urge incontinence managed with non-drug and drug treatments?
37. What are the different measurements taken during a urodynamic study and their normal ranges?
38. What are the potential complications associated with sling surgery for stress urinary incontinence?
39. How would you manage a case of vault prolapse in a 52-year-old woman who underwent a vaginal hysterectomy five years ago for uterovaginal prolapse?
40. How can vault prolapse be prevented during and after the initial surgical treatment?
41. Explain how pelvic organ prolapse is categorized?
42. How would you assess the treatment choices for a 27-year-old, who has given birth twice, with an elongated cervix below the vagina?

43. Explain the system used to quantify pelvic organ prolapse in women?
44. Describe what vaginal vault prolapse is?
45. Explain how vault prolapse is treated?
46. What does the POP-Q system for classifying uterovaginal prolapse entail?
47. How is vault prolapse managed?
48. Outline the POP-Q staging for vault prolapse?
49. Which techniques are used during a hysterectomy to minimize the risk of vault prolapse?
50. Explain the anatomical structures involved in supporting the pelvic organs?
51. What causes uterovaginal prolapse in women who have never given birth, and what surgical methods are used to treat it?
52. Which preventive measures against vault prolapse are implemented during a hysterectomy?
53. What surgical options are available for treating post-hysterectomy vault prolapse?
54. How is mesh used in the treatment of pelvic organ prolapse?
55. What are the advantages and disadvantages of using mesh in surgical procedures?
56. How are surgical meshes categorized?
57. What are the key aspects of preoperative assessment aimed at preventing post-hysterectomy vaginal vault prolapse?
58. What steps are taken during surgery to prevent post-hysterectomy vaginal vault prolapse?
59. What surgical treatments are available for vault prolapse?
60. Explain the POP-Q system for classifying pelvic organ prolapse?
61. Explain the principle behind site-specific repair for genital prolapse?
62. What strategies can be used to prevent vault prolapse?
63. What leads to a uterine prolapse, how is it categorized, and what are its signs?

64. How would you approach the treatment of vault prolapse in a 61-year-old woman?

65. Explain the anatomical structures that provide support to the pelvic organs?

66. What causes pelvic organ prolapse in a 32-year-old woman?

67. Explain the fundamental principles behind the surgical repair of an enterocele?

68. What preoperative steps should be taken before undergoing major gynecological surgery for utero-vaginal prolapse?

69. How would you provide preoperative counseling to a woman undergoing surgical treatment for uterovaginal prolapse?

70. How would you approach the management of a bladder injury encountered during the repair of a cystocele?

71. Describe the measurement system used for assessing pelvic organ prolapse known as POP-Q (Pelvic Organ Prolapse Quantification).

72. How does the POP-Q (Pelvic Organ Prolapse Quantification) system compare to traditional staging systems used for assessing pelvic organ prolapse?

73. Examine the universal applicability of the POP-Q (Pelvic Organ Prolapse Quantification) system from a critical perspective.

74. What are the strategies to prevent ureteric injuries during endoscopic surgical procedures?

75. How would you approach the treatment of an ureterovaginal fistula following a hysterectomy?

76. Discuss the clinical scenario of a urinary leak per vaginum occurring on the fifth post-operative day following an abdominal hysterectomy.

77. Outline the steps involved in establishing a management plan for a patient experiencing a urinary leak per vaginum on the fifth day post-abdominal hysterectomy.

78. Enumerate the factors that correlate with an elevated likelihood of urinary tract injuries.

79. Explain the measures taken to prevent urinary tract injuries during hysterectomy.

80. List the various factors that contribute to the development of genitourinary fistulas.
81. Outline the fundamental principles guiding the management of a fistula occurring after hysterectomy.
82. List the potential complications associated with female sterilization procedures.
83. List the etiological factors contributing to the development of vesicovaginal fistulas.
84. Discuss the fundamental principles underlying the management of vesicovaginal fistulas.
85. List the various treatment modalities available for radiation-induced fistulas.
86. Detail the preoperative assessment process for vesicovaginal fistula.
87. Outline the surgical principles involved in managing vesicovaginal fistulas occurring post-hysterectomy.
88. Outline the steps involved in the postoperative management of vesicovaginal fistula.

INFERTILITY

1. What are the potential factors contributing to male infertility?
2. Discuss the assessment and treatment of tubal factor infertility.
3. Explain how to interpret and address abnormal findings in a semen analysis report.
4. What is the meaning of the term azoospermia and its type?
5. What is Sperm retrieval technique?
6. What are the criteria used to determine normal parameters in a semen analysis according to the World Health Organization (WHO)?
7. Could you outline the diagnostic process for evaluating individuals presenting with azoospermia?
8. Describe the diagnostic approach for assessing a male partner presenting with oligospermia?
9. What is the procedure and purpose of intrauterine insemination (IUI)?

10. What are the methods used to obtain sperm for assisted reproductive techniques?
11. Describe the process for evaluating a semen sample in a laboratory setting.
12. What are the available treatment options for addressing male infertility?
13. What are the criteria or conditions that make a patient a suitable candidate for intrauterine insemination (IUI)?
14. Provide an overview of the various techniques used for preparing semen samples for assisted reproductive procedures?
15. What are factors or conditions that can contribute to male infertility?
16. Outline the typical parameters used to assess semen quality in a reproductive health context?
17. Describe the approach you would take to address infertility in a couple where the male partner has oligospermia.
18. Outline the potential causes or reasons behind secondary infertility
19. Provide guidance on the management of secondary infertility in a couple, both 32 years old, married for 8 years, experiencing infertility for 6 years following 2 previous abortions, and with no living children?
20. What diagnostic methods are available for assessing ovulation?
21. Define ovarian hyperstimulation syndrome
22. What are the diagnostic criteria and treatment strategies for ovarian hyperstimulation syndrome (OHSS)?
23. How can we effectively prevent Ovarian Hyperstimulation Syndrome (OHSS)?
24. What is Ovulation Induction and How Does it Work?
25. Mention common protocols used for inducing ovulation.
26. Discuss strategies for preventing and managing ovarian hyperstimulation syndrome.
27. How is Ovarian Hyperstimulation Syndrome (OHSS) typically handled?
28. How is the process of regulating ovarian stimulation and tracking follicle development usually described or overseen?

29. How might you address the case of a 33-year-old woman with PCOS who has successfully conceived through IVF, but shortly after embryo transfer, she arrives at the emergency department complaining of nausea, vomiting, difficulty breathing, and abdominal discomfort?
30. What is the diagnosis of above case?
31. Give an outline of your management plan of above case.
32. What measures can be taken to prevent this complication?
33. How do you facilitate ovulation in individuals with PCOS?
34. How can ovarian hyperstimulation syndrome (OHSS) be prevented and handled?
35. What are the utero-tubal and peritoneal factors affecting infertility in women?
36. What is the role of hysteroscopic surgery in treating infertility?
37. How are tubal factors assessed in cases of infertility?
38. What is the significance of tubal clipping in hydrosalpinx treatment before undergoing IVF?
39. What is the significance of tubal recanalization in the context of contemporary fertility treatments?
40. What is the significance of surgical interventions for addressing infertility due to tubal factors?
41. How is unexplained infertility treated?
42. What are the potential reasons and diagnostic approaches for a 31-year-old woman who has experienced two miscarriages and is facing challenges conceiving?
43. What strategies are employed to address blocked fallopian tubes?
44. How can the risk of multiple pregnancies be reduced in treatments using assisted reproductive technologies?
45. What is fetal reduction?
46. How Fetal Reduction Is Performed?
47. What are the reasons for and difficulties associated with choosing elective single embryo transfer (eSET)?
48. What are the various indicators used to assess ovarian reserve?
49. What are the reasons for using IVF with Intracytoplasmic Sperm Injection (ICSI)?

50. What does preimplantation genetic testing (PGT) entail?

51. What is Assisted Reproductive Technology (ART) and its complications?

52. What are the applications of Assisted Reproductive Technology (ART)?

53. What are the various stages involved in an IVF cycle?

54. What are the strategies to avoid Ovarian Hyperstimulation Syndrome (OHSS)?

55. What is the role of time-lapse imaging in monitoring embryo development within an IVF laboratory?

56. How is embryo quality evaluated in Assisted Reproductive Technology (ART)?

57. What are the circumstances in which surrogacy might be recommended?

58. What are the role of Cryo-freezing in Assisted Reproductive Technology?

59. What are the risk factors of Assisted Reproductive Technology?

60. What techniques are encompassed by Assisted Reproductive Technology (ART)?

61. What are the recent guidelines for ART?

62. What is your perspective on pre-implantation genetic diagnosis?

63. Define infertility that has no identified cause.

64. What is the significance of laparoscopy and hysteroscopy in treating women who have infertility without a known cause?

65. 11. How would you approach the treatment of a woman with infertility of unknown origin?

66. What causes infertility in cases of genital tuberculosis?

67. What is the significance of minimally invasive surgical techniques in treating endometriosis?

68. How do you approach the treatment of endometriomas in young women who are infertile?

69. What are the underlying mechanisms that lead to infertility in individuals with endometriosis?

70. Assess the pros and cons of different therapeutic approaches for young women with endometriosis.
71. How does mild endometriosis affect a woman's ability to conceive?
72. What methods can increase the likelihood of conceiving for individuals with mild endometriosis?
73. What insights or information have you acquired from the discussion, activity, assignment, or evaluation?
74. Discuss the techniques for freezing embryos and egg cells, and how long they can be effectively stored.
75. What factors affect the success rates of achieving a pregnancy using frozen embryos or egg cells?
76. Discuss the freezing and storage of ovarian tissue.
77. What does surrogacy entail, and for what medical reasons is it recommended?
78. What are the ethical concerns associated with the Surrogacy Bill?
79. What are the key elements of 'The Surrogacy (Regulation) Act, 2021'?
80. What are the issues associated with commercial surrogacy?
81. What are the drawbacks of 'The Surrogacy (Regulation) Act, 2021'?
82. What steps are involved in obtaining consent and preparing a surrogate for IVF-ET?
83. What are the markers used to evaluate ovarian reserve?
84. Explain the function and structure of the hypothalamic-pituitary-ovarian (HPO) axis?
85. What are the treatment options for infertility due to hypogonadotropic hypoestrogenism?
86. What are the causes of Hyperprolactinemia and its management?
87. What is Luteinizing Hormone (LH) surge and its functions?
88. What are the signs of an Luteinizing Hormone (LH) surge?
89. What are the methods of ovulation trigger?
90. What is ovarian reserve and its role in infertility?

91. Outline the management strategies for a woman with infertility who has a poor response to ovarian stimulation.
92. What methods are available to assess ovarian reserve?
93. What is the importance of measuring Anti-Müllerian Hormone (AMH) levels?
94. How does the endometrium change throughout the menstrual cycle?
95. What does the term Uterine Biophysical Profile (UBP) refer to?
96. How do ultrasound and color Doppler contribute to assessing the uterine environment?

MENOPAUSE

1. What is Genitourinary syndrome of menopause?
2. What are its symptoms?
3. How does it affect the quality of life of a postmenopausal woman?
4. Discuss the current status of hormonal and nonhormonal treatments for it?
5. What factors contribute to the occurrence of postmenopausal bleeding?
6. How would you approach the management of a 60-year-old woman presenting with a malodorous discharge and bleeding after intercourse?
7. What are the typical signs and how is menopause diagnosed?
8. Provide a concise definition of menopause?
9. What is definition of osteoporosis?
10. How can post-menopausal osteoporosis be prevented?
11. How is post-menopausal osteoporosis diagnosed and managed?
12. What are the hormonal changes that occur during the climacteric phase and menopause?
13. What role does hormone therapy play in addressing genitourinary symptoms in postmenopausal women?
14. What screening tests and health advice do you suggest for postmenopausal women?

15. What are the current perspectives on hormonal therapy for managing menopausal symptoms and associated health risks in postmenopausal women?
16. What are the common symptoms associated with menopause?
17. What are the treatment options for managing vasomotor symptoms during menopause?
18. What are the key points regarding the prevention, diagnosis, and management of postmenopausal osteoporosis?
19. What are the key aspects of the current utilization of menopausal hormone therapy?
20. What is the impact of menopausal hormone therapy on gynecological malignancies in brief?
21. What are the key considerations regarding the use of menopausal hormone therapy (MHT) following a hysterectomy with bilateral salpingo-oophorectomy (BSO) for endometriosis?
22. What are the current uses and controversies surrounding Hormone Replacement Therapy (HRT)?
23. How do gynecologists contribute to preventing osteoporosis in postmenopausal women?
24. What pharmacological treatments are available for managing osteoporosis in postmenopausal women?
25. What is the role of gynecologists in preventing osteoporosis in postmenopausal women?
26. What drugs can be used in preventing osteoporosis in postmenopausal women
27. Define Menopause?
28. What are the menopausal symptoms?
29. What are the treatment options for managing vasomotor symptoms associated with menopause?
30. Preventive measures for postmenopausal osteoporosis:
31. What are the underlying mechanisms contributing to osteoporosis in postmenopausal women?
32. How can postmenopausal osteoporosis be prevented, diagnosed, and managed effectively?

33. Contemporary approaches to managing menopausal symptoms.
34. Role of menopausal hormone therapy in gynecological malignancies
35. What is the role of menopausal hormone therapy in managing symptoms and potential health risks following a hysterectomy with bilateral salpingo-oophorectomy (BSO) for endometriosis?
36. What are the current medical indications for hormone replacement therapy (HRT), and what are the associated controversies? Current indications of HRT and the controversies.
37. What is the role of gynecologists in preventing osteoporosis in postmenopausal women?
38. What pharmacological treatments are available for managing osteoporosis?
39. What is the current role of hormone replacement therapy (HRT) in clinical practice?
40. What factors influence bone health in postmenopausal women?
41. What are the preventive measures for reducing the risk of osteoporosis in postmenopausal women?
42. What diagnostic methods are used to identify postmenopausal osteoporosis?
43. What is peri-menopausal transition?
44. What are the management of hot flushes in menopausal?
45. What are the role of local oestrogen therapy in a menopausal woman?

LABOUR

1. What are some factors contributing to shoulder dystocia during childbirth?
2. What diagnostic methods are used to identify shoulder dystocia during labor?
3. What potential adverse outcomes can arise from shoulder dystocia?
4. What are the strategies and procedures employed to address shoulder dystocia during labor?
5. What factors contribute to the prediction of shoulder dystocia risk?

6. What maternal and fetal complications can arise from shoulder dystocia?
7. What factors increase the likelihood of shoulder dystocia occurring?
8. What are the key recommendations for the management of shoulder dystocia cases?
9. Enumerate the potential complications experienced by mothers and newborns due to shoulder dystocia.
10. What is meant by the term 'trial of labor'?
11. What are the criteria or circumstances that warrant a trial of labor?
12. What factors contribute to favorable or unfavorable outcomes during a trial of labor?
13. How is a trial of labor typically managed or carried out?
14. What does the acronym VBAC stand for?
15. What factors contribute to the likelihood of a successful VBAC (Vaginal Birth After Cesarean)?
16. What conditions or criteria must be met for a woman to be considered eligible for Vaginal Birth After Cesarean (VBAC)?
17. What information and guidance would you provide to a patient considering Vaginal Birth After Cesarean (VBAC)?
18. How do you conduct monitoring for a patient with a history of previous Cesarean section during labor?
19. What approaches can be implemented to decrease the incidence of cesarean sections?
20. What is the Robson classification system used for?
21. What are some of the common factors that lead to an increase in cesarean section rates?
22. How do you approach counseling for pregnant women who express a preference for elective cesarean delivery?
23. What are the advantages and disadvantages associated with elective cesarean section upon request?
24. What are the potential health concerns for newborns born via elective cesarean section?
25. What is meant by the term 'cesarean scar pregnancy'?

26. What is meant by the term 'induction of labor'?
27. What distiguishes between augmentation and induction of labor?
28. What factors need to be considered before proceeding with induction of labor?
29. What are the different approaches or techniques used for induction of labor (IOL)?
30. What are the benefits associated with active management of labor (AMOL)?
31. What are the various techniques utilized to initiate or enhance labor?
32. What factors are indicative of a higher likelihood of successful labor induction?
33. What factors contribute to cervical tears during childbirth?
34. What are the signs and diagnostic procedures used to identify a cervical tear during delivery?
35. What treatment approaches are recommended for managing a case of cervical tear during childbirth?
36. What types of injuries can occur during childbirth?
37. How can you predict and mitigate the risk of birth injuries?
38. Describe the diagnostic process and management strategies for a primigravida patient at 41 weeks and 2 days of gestational age who has not yet entered labor.
39. What considerations are involved in interpreting abnormal cardiotocography (CTG) results?
40. What is the definition of a partogram?
41. What updates or revisions have been made in the most recent labor care guidelines released by the World Health Organization (WHO)?
42. What methods are utilized for intrapartum fetal monitoring in pregnancies deemed high risk?
43. How does intrauterine resuscitation contribute to managing cases of intrapartum fetal distress?
44. What is involved in the process of intrapartum fetal monitoring?
45. What circumstances warrant the use of electronic fetal monitoring (EFM)?

46. What factors can lead to fetal bradycardia and tachycardia during labor?
47. What approaches are typically employed to address late decelerations during labor?
48. What assessments are typically conducted when a woman enters the onset of labor?
49. What are the various techniques used for monitoring the fetus during labor?
50. What distinguishes between a normal and abnormal tracing observed during electronic fetal monitoring?
51. What does the term 'active management' refer to in the context of the third stage of labor?
52. What are the surgical procedures used to address postpartum hemorrhage resulting from uterine atony?
53. What does active management involve during the third stage of labor?
54. What is the significance of the lower uterine segment in pregnancy and childbirth?
55. What are the signs and symptoms indicative of obstructed labor due to cephalopelvic disproportion (CPD)?
56. What challenges may be encountered during the second stage of a cesarean section (SSCS)?
57. How is the delivery of the second twin typically managed during childbirth?
58. What is meant by the term 'embryo reduction'?
59. What is meant by the term 'active phase' during labor?
60. What are the abnormalities that can occur during the active phase of labor, and how are they managed?
61. Explain the significance and function of epidural analgesia during the process of childbirth.
62. Explain the advantages and disadvantages of delivering a baby in a water environment.
63. Illustrate the benefits and drawbacks of utilizing morphine as a pain management option during labor.

64. List the various approaches available for providing pain relief during childbirth.

65. Identify situations where neuraxial analgesia may not be advisable or suitable.

66. Discuss strategies for managing headaches resulting from post-dural puncture, including its causes and treatment options.

67. Explain the concept and procedure of external cephalic version.

68. Outline the necessary conditions and potential risks associated with external cephalic version.

69. List factors that can contribute to a fetus being in the breech presentation position during pregnancy.

70. Examine the available strategies for managing breech presentation in a woman with multiple pregnancies at full term.

71. Describe the techniques utilized for delivering the after-coming head during breech presentations.

72. Discuss the approach to handling a shoulder presentation that has been neglected or undiagnosed until delivery.

73. Explore the procedures involved in managing the delivery of the head following a breech presentation.

74. Discuss the precautionary measures necessary during the delivery of a premature baby in the breech presentation position.

75. Examine the occipito-posterior fetal position during labor and its management, with a focus on delivering the baby's face to the pubis.

76. A woman who has had multiple pregnancies and is at full term presents with a fetus in a transverse lie position.

77. Which diagnostic tests or examinations would you recommend, and what are the reasons for their necessity?

78. What steps would you take to address her condition and provide appropriate care?

79. Enumerate the factors that increase the likelihood of a breech presentation during pregnancy.

80. What steps would you take to address the situation if a similar case presents at 36 weeks of gestation?

81. Enumerate the factors contributing to fetal malpresentations during the final stages of pregnancy.
82. List the obstetric complications associated with fetal malpresentations during childbirth.
83. Explain the contemporary recommendations and procedures for external cephalic version according to current medical guidelines and protocols.
84. Enumerate the circumstances or conditions that warrant the initiation of labor induction.
85. List the components of the Bishop's score and discuss its relevance in assessing the readiness for labor induction.
86. Outline various techniques for labor induction and emphasize the method and applications of oxytocin in this process.

Chapter - 3

REPRODUCTIVE ENDOCRINOLOGY

1. What are the causes of primary amenorrhea?
2. What is the management approach for an 18-year-old with androgen insensitivity syndrome?
3. How is primary amenorrhea methodically evaluated and diagnosed?
4. What is Turner syndrome?
5. What is secondary amenorrhea?
6. How about we explore creating a management flow chart for a case of secondary amenorrhea?
7. What are the key factors necessary for the initiation and maintenance of regular menstrual cycles?
8. What are the causes of crypto-menorrhea?
9. How would you assess a 16-year-old girl who has not yet started menstruating?
10. What are the reasons for the occurrence of secondary amenorrhea?
11. What is the approach to assessing a 30-year-old woman who has experienced secondary amenorrhea since her last childbirth five years ago?
12. What defines the syndrome characterized by the presence of galactorrhea and amenorrhea?
13. What are the key strategies for treating galactorrhea-amenorrhea in a 23-year-old female?
14. How is gender dysphoria defined in adolescents?
15. What are the challenges and approaches to care for transgender adolescents?
16. How are ovulatory disorders categorized?

17. How is anovulation treated in a 31-year-old female?
18. How should a 21-year-old woman presenting with hirsutism be evaluated?
19. Summarize the guidelines recommended by the Endocrine Society
20. What steps should be taken to evaluate and manage a 26-year-old unmarried woman who presents to the gynecology clinic with excessive facial hair growth?
21. What are the common drugs used for treatment of hirsutism and their side effects of these drugs?
22. What are the established criteria for diagnosing Polycystic Ovary Syndrome (PCOS)?
23. How should polycystic ovary syndrome (PCOS) be managed in adolescent females?
24. What steps are involved in diagnosing polycystic ovary syndrome (PCOS) in adolescents?
25. What are the methods to stimulate ovulation in individuals with polycystic ovary syndrome (PCOS)?
26. How can ovarian hyperstimulation syndrome be prevented and managed?
27. What are the biochemical and endocrinological characteristics of young women with PCOS, and how do these factors influence infertility?
28. What could be the tentative diagnosis for an 18-year-old girl presenting with obesity and infrequent menstrual periods?
29. What diagnostic tests should be performed for evaluating obesity and infrequent menstrual periods, and what management strategies are recommended?
30. What is the definition of precocious puberty, and what are its potential causes?
31. How should precocious puberty be managed in a 7-year-old girl?
32. Understanding the Physical Transformations During Puberty.
33. What are the hormonal and physical transformations that occur during puberty?

34. What triggers the early onset of puberty?
35. What is the clinical evaluation strategy for delayed puberty in an adolescent girl?
36. What are the possible diagnoses for a delayed onset of puberty?
37. What diagnostic approach would you take for a 17-year-old girl experiencing delayed puberty?
38. What is the order of changes that occur during puberty?
39. How would you approach the evaluation and management of iron deficiency anemia in adolescent girls?
40. What are the differential diagnosis of delayed pubertal development?
41. What investigations would you conduct for a 17-year-old girl with delayed pubertal development?
42. What is the sequence of pubertal changes?
43. What are the causes of heavy menstrual bleeding during puberty?
44. How is heavy menstrual bleeding during puberty managed?
45. What are the differential diagnoses for heavy menstrual bleeding during puberty?
46. What are the diagnostic criteria for Premature Ovarian Insufficiency (POI)?
47. How is Premature Ovarian Insufficiency (POI) evaluated and managed?
48. What are the different tests used to assess ovarian reserve?
49. What are the different causes of premature ovarian failure (POF)?
50. What are the long-term clinical implications of premature ovarian failure (POF)?
51. What causes primary ovarian insufficiency (POI)?
52. What is premature ovarian failure (POF)?
53. What are the causes, consequences, and health impacts of premature ovarian failure (POF)?
54. What methods are used to diagnose and manage premature ovarian failure (POF)?
55. What are the different methods used to evaluate ovarian reserve?

56. What are the causes of ovarian failure not related to chromosomal abnormalities?
57. What strategies are used to manage premature ovarian failure in a 23-year-old woman?
58. What leads to the development of premature ovarian failure (POF)?
59. What is the approach to evaluating a case of premature ovarian failure (POF)?
60. What are the treatment options and management strategies for a case of premature ovarian failure (POF) accompanied by infertility?
61. What are the types of Müllerian duct anomalies?
62. What are the health complications linked to Müllerian duct anomalies?
63. What is the approach to treating hematocolpos due to a transverse vaginal septum in an adolescent?
64. What is the brief overview of the embryonic development of the female reproductive system?
65. What are the methods for diagnosing and treating a bicornuate uterus?
66. How does the Müllerian duct develop?
67. What is the role of anti-Müllerian hormone in development?
68. What is the updated classification for congenital uterine anomalies?
69. What are the approaches to managing hysteroscopic septal resection and its potential complications?
70. What are the classifications of Müllerian duct anomalies?
71. What are the methods used to diagnose different Müllerian duct anomalies?
72. How are Müllerian duct anomalies classified and what renal tract abnormalities are associated with them?
73. What approach is taken to diagnose and treat cryptomenorrhea?
74. What is the current classification system for Müllerian agenesis?
75. How is vaginoplasty used in the treatment of Müllerian agenesis?
76. What are the management strategies for a patient with Complete Androgen Insensitivity Syndrome (CAIS)?

77. What is the classification system for Müllerian abnormalities?
78. What are the reproductive challenges faced by women with Müllerian abnormalities and how are they managed?
79. How do you approach the diagnosis and management of pubertal disorders in young girls?
80. What are the types of Müllerian anomalies, and what is their importance in Obstetrics and Gynecology?
81. What are the strategies for diagnosing and treating an intrauterine septum?
82. What are the categories of Müllerian duct anomalies and their associated clinical symptoms?
83. What is the approach to treating hematocolpos due to a transverse vaginal septum in an adolescent girl?
84. How can you illustrate the various Müllerian duct anomalies through diagrams?
85. What are the gynecological and obstetric complications associated with Müllerian duct anomalies?
86. What is the management strategy for a septate uterus?

HIV

1. Explain briefly post-exposure prophylaxis for HIV?
2. How does HIV infection impact a pregnancy?
3. How should the antenatal care be managed for a 32-year-old pregnant woman, at 12 weeks gestation, who has tested positive for HIV?
4. What are the current guidelines for the treatment of pregnant women who are HIV positive?
5. What are the current national guidelines for antenatal care to prevent vertical transmission of HIV from mother to newborn?
6. What are the current national guidelines for the follow-up care of a neonate born to an HIV seropositive mother?
7. What are the current WHO guidelines for managing neonates born to HIV-infected mothers?

8. What are the details of management during labor and after delivery?
9. What are the four critical elements involved in preventing HIV transmission from a pregnant woman to her baby?
10. What are the guidelines for breastfeeding and newborn prophylaxis in the context of HIV?
11. What are the guidelines for managing the delivery of HIV-positive women and their newborns?
12. What are the latest guidelines for breastfeeding among HIV-positive women in developing countries?
13. What does vertical transmission refer to?
14. What factors affect the perinatal transmission of HIV and how can it be prevented?
15. What factors increase the risk of transmitting HIV?
16. What is the typical progression of HIV infection in humans?
17. What methods are used to prevent the vertical transmission of HIV from a mother to her baby?
18. What strategies are employed to prevent perinatal transmission of HIV in pregnant women?
19. What strategies are recommended for managing a newborn whose mother is HIV positive?
20. What strategies are used to prevent the transmission of HIV from parent to child?
21. What types of HIV testing are recommended for pregnant women?

Chapter - 4

MEDICAL TERMINATION OF PREGNANCY

1. How can one approach and perform a medical termination of pregnancy during the first trimester?
2. What are the key provisions and implications of the Medical Termination of Pregnancy Act?
3. What are the recommended treatment approaches for septic abortion?
4. Explain the procedures commonly used for terminating a pregnancy during the second trimester?
5. Considering a scenario where Mifepristone and Misoprostol were administered as per protocol for a patient undergoing medical termination of pregnancy at 18 weeks, yet the desired outcome wasn't achieved. Explore the potential factors contributing to this outcome and propose appropriate management strategies for the case.
6. Elaborate on the concept of the 'cafeteria approach' in post-abortion contraception counseling?
7. Discuss the considerations regarding the timing of initiation, along with the associated pros and cons?
8. What are the key modifications or revisions made to the initial Medical Termination of Pregnancy (MTP) Act?
9. What are the provisions and significance of the Medical Termination of Pregnancy (MTP) Act of 1971.
10. Outline the criteria or circumstances that warrant termination of pregnancy as per the provisions of this Act?
11. Enumerate the different techniques utilized for terminating pregnancy during the first trimester?

12. List the benefits and drawbacks associated with medical methods of abortion?
13. What are the potential adverse outcomes or risks associated with manual vacuum aspiration?

NEONATOLOGY

1. Explain the concept and components of initiatives promoting a "baby-friendly" hospital environment.
2. Examine the practice and benefits of Kangaroo Mother Care.
3. Outline the approach to managing a neonate with Rh isoimmunization.
4. Discuss the benefits and drawbacks of antenatal corticosteroid therapy.
5. Explain the different medications, dosages, and guidelines for antenatal corticosteroid therapy.
6. Examine the care and interventions required for a neonate born to a mother with HIV infection.
7. Explore methods for diagnosing and preventing early-onset neonatal sepsis.
8. Explain the principles and practice of Kangaroo Mother Care.
9. Discuss the protocols and techniques involved in neonatal resuscitation.
10. Define neonatal sepsis and categorize its types.
11. Detail the therapeutic approach for addressing neonatal sepsis.
12. Explain the significance and components of the Apgar score.
13. Discuss the use and implications of antenatal corticosteroids.
14. Distinguish between caput succedaneum, subgaleal hematoma, and cephalohematoma.
15. Explore the etiology and therapeutic approaches for caput succedaneum, subgaleal hematoma, and cephalohematoma.
16. Discuss the key components of essential care for newborns.
17. Explore neonatal jaundice, its causes, and management.

18. Examine hypoxic-ischemic encephalopathy (HIE), including its etiology, clinical features, and management.
19. Define respiratory distress syndrome (RDS) and discuss its characteristics.
20. Enumerate potential causes of respiratory distress in newborns.
21. Discuss the therapeutic strategies for managing respiratory distress syndrome in newborns.
22. List congenital malformations in newborns that require urgent surgical intervention.
23. Examine the diagnostic process and therapeutic approaches for tracheoesophageal fistula.
24. Enumerate the potential etiological factors contributing to jaundice in newborns.
25. Explain the underlying reasons for implementing phototherapy in the management of neonatal hyperbilirubinemia.
26. Outline the essential care measures for newborns undergoing phototherapy.
27. Enumerate the etiological factors, clinical manifestations, and potential complications of pathological jaundice in newborns.
28. Explain the mechanism by which exchange transfusion benefits a neonate with Rh isoimmunization.
29. Describe the cardiopulmonary adaptations that occur in a newborn infant.
30. Create a flowchart outlining the sequential steps of neonatal resuscitation
31. Enumerate eight maternal conditions that necessitate the presence of a neonatal resuscitation team during delivery.
32. Outline the approach to caring for a newborn born to a mother with diabetes.
33. Discuss the management of a newborn born to an Rh-negative mother.
34. Examine the care protocol for a newborn born to an HIV-positive mother.

35. Discuss the approach to caring for a newborn born to a mother with epilepsy.
36. Examine the care plan for a newborn born to a mother who is positive for beta thalassemia trait.
37. What is meant by birth asphyxia?
38. Explaining the concept of a modified biophysical profile score.
39. Discuss the significance and purpose of the admission test.
40. Outline the potential neonatal complications associated with infants born to diabetic mothers.
41. Describe the physiological process of the initiation of air breathing in the newborn following delivery.
42. What methods are used to assess the condition of a newborn?
43. Outline the fundamental resuscitation procedures for a newborn in the delivery room.
44. Describe the assessment process used to evaluate the condition of a newborn immediately after birth.
45. Outline the step-by-step algorithm for the resuscitation protocol in newborns.
46. Discuss respiratory distress syndrome (RDS) in newborns, including its definition, etiology, and preventive measures.
47. Define cephalohematoma and elucidate its characteristics.
48. Explain the causes and therapeutic approaches for cephalo-hematoma.
49. Enumerate the factors contributing to neonatal jaundice.
50. Examine kernicterus briefly and discuss the role of phototherapy in its management.
51. Outline the key components of neonatal resuscitation.
52. Examine the therapeutic approach for managing neonatal hypoglycemia.
53. Explore the advantages of breastfeeding for both the mother and newborn.
54. Examine the processes of galactogenesis and lactogenesis.
55. Define birth asphyxia and elucidate its implications.

56. Discuss preventive measures to mitigate the risk of birth asphyxia in growth-restricted infants
57. List the potential long-term consequences of birth asphyxia.
58. Provide a brief overview of hypoxic-ischemic encephalopathy.
59. Provide a concise explanation of neonatal jaundice.
60. Enumerate the factors contributing to fetal anemia.
61. Outline the diagnostic techniques employed for detecting fetal anemia.
62. Discuss the treatment strategies for managing fetal anemia.
63. Explain the significance and components of the APGAR score.
64. Outline the resuscitation procedures for a newborn with a low APGAR score.
65. Define birth asphyxia and list its immediate and long-term consequences.

FETAL MEDICINE

1. Explore non-invasive methods used in prenatal care to detect fetal anomalies.
2. Examine the diverse intrauterine fetal therapies available, including their indications and procedural details.
3. What does the term 'Ex-utero Intrafetal Treatment procedure (EXIT)' refer to?
4. What constitutes fetal therapy?
5. Examine the principles, indications, and classification of fetal therapy.
6. Enumerate the various approaches to fetal therapy.
7. Explain the procedure known as EXIT surgery?
8. Elaborate on the presence of cystic hygroma observed during a fetal anomaly scan?
9. What implications might the detection of liver calcification in a primigravida fetus at 19 weeks of gestation have based on ultrasound findings?

10. Examine the factors contributing to fetal liver calcification.
11. What approaches would you consider for addressing this case?
12. Explore the implications of bilateral renal pelvicalyceal dilatation observed in a fetus of a primigravida who conceived via in-vitro fertilization after a prolonged period of infertility, at 24 weeks of gestation?
13. Delve into the potential factors contributing to bilateral renal pelvicalyceal dilatation in this scenario?
14. What strategies would you consider for the management of this case?
15. Elaborate on the purposes and significance of fetal MRI in clinical practice?
16. What are the biochemical indicators utilized to identify fetal anomalies during the first trimester of pregnancy?
17. How is congenital diaphragmatic hernia detected prenatally?
18. How does the presence of echogenic bowel appear on antenatal ultrasonography, and what implications might it have?
19. What contributions does MRI make to obstetrics and gynecology?

ULTRASONOGRAPHY

1. How does uterine artery embolization play a role in managing abnormal uterine bleeding?
2. How does Doppler velocimetry contribute to evaluating placental circulation?
3. What are the clinical applications of Doppler velocimetry in pregnancy?
4. What safety guidelines should be followed for imaging modalities during pregnancy?
5. Provide an overview of the indications, procedure, and potential complications associated with uterine artery embolization?
6. In what ways does sonography enhance aneuploidy screening?
7. What are the soft signs commonly associated with fetal trisomy 21?

8. What methods are available for determining chorionicity during pregnancy?
9. How does chorionicity impact the management of twin pregnancy?
10. How does imaging contribute to the diagnosis and management of adenomyosis?
11. Discuss the utilization of Doppler studies in gynecological cases.
12. How does transvaginal ultrasound (TVS) contribute to the investigation and management of infertility?
13. How does ultrasonography play a role in assessing and managing infertility?
14. What is the significance of uterine artery Doppler studies during pregnancy?
15. What are the recommended guidelines for measuring nuchal translucency during first-trimester fetal anomaly screening?
16. What constitutes the standard examination of fetal anatomy during a second-trimester anomaly scan?
17. What is the clinical significance of Doppler studies in fetal growth restriction?
18. What perinatal complications can arise in cases of fetal growth restriction? Outline their management strategies.
19. What are the fundamental principles underlying the assessment of fetal ductus venosus flow?
20. What distinguishable features characterize normal and abnormal waveforms in fetal ductus venosus flow assessment?
21. What are the clinical situations that warrant the utilization of fetal ductus venosus flow assessment?
22. In what ways does fetal ductus venosus flow assessment influence obstetric management?
23. What elements comprise a typical ultrasound examination during the first and second trimesters of pregnancy?
24. What are the established guidelines for measuring nuchal translucency thickness?

25. What are the potential abnormalities encountered when measuring the biparietal diameter?
26. Which fetal anatomical parameters should be assessed during a second-trimester fetal anomaly detection scan?
27. What are the types of neural tube defects that can occur in a fetus?
28. What is the recommended approach for managing a subsequent pregnancy in a woman with a history of a fetus affected by a neural tube defect?
29. What is Doppler flow velocimetry, and how does it contribute to the management of pregnancy?
30. What are the situations in obstetrics where MRI is indicated?
31. What is the clinical significance of the presence of a yolk sac within the gestational sac in obstetrics?
32. How does ultrasound play a role in managing mono-chorionic twin pregnancies?
33. What is the role of sonography in the first trimester of pregnancy?
34. Elaborate on soft markers used to indicate the possibility of fetal aneuploidy?
35. What is meant by MCA-PSV (Middle Cerebral Artery Peak Systolic Velocity)?
36. How does MCA-PSV (Middle Cerebral Artery Peak Systolic Velocity) contribute to obstetrics?
37. Provide a brief overview of the clinical significance of Doppler studies in obstetrics?
38. Briefly explain the underlying principles of Doppler velocimetry?
39. What are the major vessels examined during pregnancy via Doppler velocimetry, and how do their assessments influence pregnancy management?
40. How do Doppler studies prove useful in cases of multiple gestation?
41. How do Doppler studies prove useful in assessing infertility in women?
42. How are Doppler studies utilized in cases of placenta previa?

ENDOSCOPY

1. What is the role of Natural Orifice Transluminal Endoscopic Surgery (NOTES) in Obstetrics and Gynecology?
2. How does ergonomics factor into endoscopic surgery?
3. What are the fundamental principles governing the use of an electrosurgical unit in gynecological surgery?
4. How does minimally invasive surgery contribute to the management of endometriosis?
5. Elaborate on the approach to managing recurrent endometriosis in cases of infertility?
6. What are the perioperative complications associated with electrosurgery in laparoscopic surgeries, and how can they be prevented?
7. How does hysteroscopy contribute to the diagnosis and management of gynecological conditions?
8. What are the potential complications associated with hysteroscopy?
9. What are the preventive measures to reduce the risk of complications during hysteroscopy?
10. What is the procedure for conducting a hysteroscopy in an office setting?
11. What are the indications, prerequisites, and precautions for an office hysteroscopy?
12. How are endometrial polyps managed during a hysteroscopy?
13. What is the role of robotic surgery in gynecology?
14. What is the significance of interventional radiology in gynecology?
15. What is the significance of laparoscopy in gynecology?
16. How are different energy sources evaluated for hemostasis in endoscopic surgery?
17. What are the benefits of using robotic surgery?
18. How does hysteroscopy contribute to the management of infertility?
19. What are the indications and potential complications of laparoscopic surgery?

20. What distinguishes robotic surgery from laparoscopic surgery, and what is its role in gynecology?
21. What are the indications and potential complications associated with hysteroscopy?
22. What are the strategies for managing complications arising from hysteroscopy?
23. What preparations are required before undergoing laparoscopic surgery?
24. What are the indications for and potential complications of laparoscopic surgery in gynecology?
25. What measures can be taken to prevent complications in laparoscopic surgery?
26. What are the causes of intrauterine adhesions?
27. What are the clinical consequences of intrauterine adhesions?
28. How are intrauterine adhesions managed hysteroscopically, and how can their recurrence be prevented?
29. What are the fundamental principles guiding the application of electrosurgical energy during surgical procedures?
30. Compare and contrast the advantages and disadvantages of monopolar and bipolar diathermy in surgical settings.
31. Outline the indications, procedural steps, and potential complications associated with ovarian drilling as a treatment option for polycystic ovarian syndrome.
32. What conditions warrant the use of operative laparoscopy?
33. What potential complications may arise from operative laparoscopy?
34. What strategies can be employed to anticipate and prevent complications associated with operative laparoscopy?

Chapter - 5

PHARMACOLOGY

1. How are antenatal corticosteroids administered during pregnancy, and what are the recommended dosages and guidelines for their use?
2. Provide an overview of different antihypertensive medications used during pregnancy, detailing their recommended dosages and potential side effects?
3. What is the preferred antihypertensive medication for a lactating mother in the postpartum period?
4. What information can you provide about Ulipristal acetate?
5. How effective and appropriate are the WHO Medical eligibility criteria for the use of injection medroxyprogesterone acetate as a contraceptive method?
6. What is the definition and function of selective progesterone receptor modulators?
7. What are the practical applications of selective estrogen receptor modulators (SERMs) in treating gynecological disorders?
8. Provide information about Mifepristone?
9. How do GnRH agonists and antagonists function?
10. What are the medical indications for GnRH agonists in clinical practice?
11. What is the FDA's stance regarding the use of medications during pregnancy?
12. What are the potential maternal and fetal effects associated with the use of antibacterial antibiotics during pregnancy?
13. How do the physiological changes associated with pregnancy affect the pharmacokinetics of antimicrobial medications?

14. What information can you provide about Dinogest?
15. What are GnRH antagonists?
16. What is a selective progesterone receptor modulator?
17. What methods are used to assess ovarian reserve?
18. What is the function of Atosiban in obstetrics
19. What is the significance of inositol?
20. What is the physiological function of inositol, and how does it relate to the clinical management of polycystic ovary syndrome (PCOS)?
21. What is the efficacy and safety profile of ulipristal acetate?
22. How are fibroids typically managed?
23. What are the options for emergency contraception?
24. What is the significance of progesterone in the management of recurrent pregnancy loss?
25. What is the neuroprotective function of antepartum magnesium sulfate?
26. What are the physiological roles of follicle-stimulating hormone (FSH)?
27. What are the medical reasons for prescribing gonadotropins in gynecological practice?
28. What are some examples of medications that inhibit gonadotropin activity?
29. What is a selective estrogen receptor modulator (SERM)?
30. What is the evidence supporting the use of progesterone in obstetrics?
31. What are the applications of low molecular weight heparin in obstetrics?
32. Provide a list of available agents, including their recommended dosages and potential side effects?
33. What is the role of oxytocin in the physiology of pregnancy?
34. What are the pharmacokinetic properties of oxytocin, and how is it therapeutically utilized during labor?

35. What are the pharmacodynamic effects of misoprostol?

36. What are the medical reasons for prescribing misoprostol in obstetrics?

37. What monitoring measures would you implement for a primigravida who has undergone induction at full term using vaginal misoprostol?

38. What is the definition of progestogens, and how are they categorized?

39. What are the common applications of progestogens in gynecological care?

Chapter - 6

PREVENTIVE AND SOCIAL MEDICINE

1. Provide an overview of government initiatives aimed at addressing anemia among pregnant women and newborns in India?
2. Outline the key principles that constitute publication ethics?
3. Categorize the various forms of academic misconduct related to improper citation and attribution?
4. Explore strategies for maintaining academic integrity and originality in writing?
5. Provide an explanation of the design and methodology involved in conducting a case-control study?
6. How about discussing the hierarchy of evidence in research methodology, categorized by the types of studies conducted?
7. How gynecologists contribute to the implementation and success of the National Adolescent Health Program (Rastriya Kishore Swasthya Karyakaram, RKSK)?
8. Could you delve into the strategies for addressing pregnancy complications and providing comprehensive care for adolescent mothers?
9. Outline the objectives and targets set by the National Health Mission for improving rural healthcare delivery?
10. Provide an overview of the objectives and initiatives under the Lakshya program?
11. Explore the key indicators used to assess the health and well-being of mothers, newborns, and children?
12. Categorize the different types of observational research methods used in epidemiological studies?

13. Outline the fundamental principles underlying randomized controlled trials (RCTs)?

14. How about discussing the components and importance of the Consolidated Standards of Reporting Trials guidelines in clinical research reporting?

15. How about exploring the various methodologies employed in scientific inquiry and investigation?

16. How can one effectively formulate a research inquiry or hypothesis?

17. How about discussing the diverse approaches and methodologies available for conducting research?

18. Outline a research proposal detailing the investigation into the efficacy of exercise in managing Gestational Diabetes Mellitus?

19. Explain the concept of random assignment in research methodology?

20. How about exploring different methods of sampling in research, focusing on randomization and providing examples for each technique?

21. How about discussing different measures used to assess fertility, along with their definitions and significance in demographic studies?

22. Provide an overview of the roles and responsibilities of Accredited Social Health Activists (ASHAs) in community healthcare delivery?

23. How about we delve into the duties and tasks typically assigned to Accredited Social Health Activists (ASHAs) in their role within community healthcare?

24. Explore the concept of applied research and its significance in addressing real-world problems or issues?

25. What are the different sampling techniques used in research, highlighting their respective methodologies and applications?

26. How can one effectively develop a hypothesis as the foundation of a research study?

27. Discuss the key elements necessary for conducting robust and scientifically sound research?

28. Explore the various categories or genres of scholarly publications in research?

29. Discuss the significance of conducting a thorough literature review in the research process?
30. Provide an overview of the objectives and initiatives under the Anaemia Mukt Bharat program aimed at addressing anemia in India?
31. Provide an overview of the objectives and strategies of the National Nutrition Mission aimed at addressing malnutrition in India?
32. How about we explore the concepts of maternal near-miss and severe acute maternal morbidity, along with their significance in obstetric care?
33. Explain the clinical criteria used to identify cases of maternal near miss in obstetric care?
34. How do longitudinal and cross-sectional studies differ in their approach to understanding behavior change over time?
35. What are the key factors to consider when determining the sample size for a therapeutic trial?
36. What criteria can you use to assess the scientific rigor and validity of a research study?
37. What are the key criteria outlined by the World Health Organization for evaluating screening programs?
38. Among gynecological cancers, which one aligns most closely with the criteria outlined by the World Health Organization for screening programs?
39. Explain the terms sensitivity, specificity, positive predictive value, negative predictive value, and confidence interval in the context of medical testing?
40. What does the term 'maternal mortality' refer to in the context of public health and obstetrics?
41. What are some of the leading causes contributing to maternal mortality in India?
42. What is the significance of conducting maternal death reviews in efforts to decrease maternal mortality rates?
43. What is the definition of maternal mortality, and what methodologies are employed to calculate it?
44. What are some of the factors contributing to maternal mortality?

45. What measures can be implemented to decrease maternal mortality rates?
46. What does perinatal mortality mean, and what methods are used to calculate it?
47. What are some of the factors contributing to perinatal mortality?
48. What are the standard assessment protocols recommended for investigating a case of stillbirth in a woman?
49. What is meant by the concept of written consent in the context of medical or research procedures?
50. What are the essential conditions or requirements for obtaining written consent in medical or research contexts?
51. What is the significance of written consent from a medico-legal perspective?
52. What is the current status of maternal mortality in India?
53. What are some of the key factors contributing to the high maternal mortality rate in India, and what strategies can be implemented to lower it?
54. What does the acronym RCH stand for in the context of healthcare?
55. What are the key elements or components of the reproductive and child health (RCH) program?
56. What strategies can be employed to ensure the successful implementation and outcomes of the RCH program?
57. What does the term Janani Shishu Suraksha Karyakram (JSSK) refer to?
58. What are the key features or components of the Janani Shishu Suraksha Karyakram (JSSK)?
59. What measures can be taken to ensure the effective implementation and success of the Janani Shishu Suraksha Karyakram (JSSK)?
60. What are the various benefits offered under the Janani Shishu Suraksha Karyakram (JSSK) scheme?
61. What is meant by a double-blind, placebo-controlled trial, and why is it considered significant in clinical research?
62. What is the concept of the Millennium Development Goals (MDGs)?

63. What is the progress report on the Millennium Development Goals (MDGs) in India?

64. What measures could be implemented to enhance the achievement of the Millennium Development Goals (MDGs)?

65. What are the different types of scientific studies, and how do they contribute to establishing evidence levels and recommendations for clinical practice?

66. What are the objectives, vision, targets, and components of the Reproductive and Child Health (RCH) program?

67. What are the distinctions between the first and second phases of the Reproductive and Child Health (RCH) program?

68. What is meant by the term 'Maternal Near Miss,' and what criteria does the World Health Organization (WHO) use to identify a patient as experiencing Maternal Near Miss?

69. What strategies can be implemented to lower maternal morbidity and mortality rates?

70. What initiatives has the Government of India undertaken to improve maternal and child health?

71. What are the key features of RCH-II, and what progress has been made under this program?

72. What role does ASHA play in providing reproductive healthcare services to women in rural areas?

FAMILY PLANNING

1. Provide an explanation of barrier methods of contraception?

2. What advantages are associated with the use of barrier contraceptives, and what is their typical failure rate?

3. How would you provide contraceptive counseling to a sexually active, unmarried 20-year-old woman seeking advice at an adolescent clinic?

4. What are the implications of missed doses in oral contraceptive use?

5. What are the additional health benefits of oral contraceptive pills (OCPs) beyond contraception?

6. Outline the contraindications and potential adverse effects associated with the combined oral contraceptive pill?
7. What medical conditions can be treated or managed using combined oral contraceptives (COCs)?
8. What are the potential side effects associated with combined oral contraceptives (COCs)?
9. What are the situations or medical conditions where the use of combined oral contraceptives (COCs) is not recommended?
10. How do combined oral contraceptives (COCs) interact with other medications?
11. What benefits do newer generation oral contraceptive pills offer compared to traditional or conventional OCPs?
12. What are the relative and absolute contraindications associated with newer generation oral contraceptive pills?
13. What are the medical criteria used to determine the suitability of different contraceptive methods for individuals?
14. What are the alternatives to oral hormonal contraception?
15. What are the different categories of oral contraceptive pills that are currently on the market?
16. What additional health benefits are associated with using oral contraceptive pills beyond contraception?
17. Provide a brief overview of combined injectable contraceptives?
18. Provide a brief explanation of postpartum intrauterine contraceptive devices (IUCDs)?
19. What methods are available for administering hormonal contraception?
20. Provide an overview of the vaginal contraceptive ring, including its uses, benefits, and drawbacks?
21. What are the additional health advantages of using hormonal contraception beyond preventing pregnancy?
22. What are the options available for emergency contraception?
23. Explain the different methods of emergency contraception?
24. Could you elaborate on how each method of emergency contraception works and what their respective failure rates are?

25. What are the different approaches to emergency contraception?
26. What are the mechanisms of action associated with each method of emergency contraception?
27. What are the potential side effects and effectiveness rates of different emergency contraception methods?
28. What are the considerations surrounding the availability of emergency contraceptives over-the-counter (OTC)?
29. What is the Pearl Index used to measure in contraceptive studies?
30. What is the WHO Medical Eligibility Criteria for contraceptive use, and how is it used in clinical practice?
31. Provide a comprehensive analysis of the various methods of emergency contraception, including their efficacy, safety, and practical considerations?
32. What contraceptive options would you consider for a sexually active 45-year-old patient seeking contraception?
33. Elaborate on the benefits and applications of the levonorgestrel intrauterine device (IUD) in the field of gynecology?
34. How would you approach the management of a 29-year-old woman who has a Copper T intrauterine contraceptive device (IUCD) inserted but cannot locate the threads after 2 months?
35. What contraceptive options would you recommend to a recently married couple who wish to delay childbirth for three years? Discuss the advantages and disadvantages of each method.
36. What are the different types of long-acting reversible contraception (LARC), and what are their indications and contraindications?
37. What steps would you take to address a case of displaced Copper T intrauterine contraceptive device?
38. What are the contraindications and potential complications associated with intrauterine contraceptive devices (IUCDs)?
39. What are the different types of contraceptive methods that do not rely on hormones?
40. What are the contraindications, mode of action, and potential complications associated with intrauterine copper devices (IUCDs)?

41. Provide information on long-acting reversible contraceptives (LARCs).
42. What are the different methods of long-acting reversible contraceptives (LARCs), along with their indications, contra-indications, risks, and potential side effects?
43. What are the alternatives to oral hormonal contraception?
44. What are the additional health benefits associated with combined oral contraceptive pills (COCPs) beyond contraception?
45. What are the benefits and drawbacks of using newer progestins for contraception?
46. What medical conditions are considered absolute contraindications for the use of hormonal contraceptives according to the WHO medical eligibility criteria?
47. How is tubal re-anastomosis performed and what are the guiding principles behind the procedure?
48. What are the benefits associated with third-generation intrauterine devices (IUDs)?
49. Discuss the relationship between combined oral contraceptives and the development of neoplasia?
50. What considerations should be taken into account when prescribing contraceptives for a woman with diabetes mellitus?
51. What are the different types of non-oral hormonal contraceptive methods available?
52. What are the medical applications of the levonorgestrel-releasing intrauterine system (LNG-IUS) beyond contraception?
53. What are the situations or medical conditions where the use of intrauterine devices (IUDs) is not recommended?
54. What are the potential outcomes associated with a pregnancy in which an intrauterine device (IUD) is retained?
55. How would you assess a case involving an intrauterine device (IUD) user who cannot see the device's thread?
56. What criteria does the World Health Organization (WHO) use to determine the medical eligibility for intrauterine contraceptive device (IUCD) use?

57. Describe the mechanism by which intrauterine contraceptive devices (IUCDs) prevent pregnancy?

58. What are the benefits and drawbacks associated with intrauterine contraceptive devices (IUCDs) that contain progesterone?

59. What initiatives has the Government of India undertaken regarding the insertion of post-placental intrauterine contraceptive devices (PP-IUCDs)?

60. What are frameless intrauterine devices (IUDs)?

61. Discuss the relationship between pelvic inflammatory disease (PID) and the use of intrauterine contraceptive devices (IUCDs)?

62. What are the different types of intrauterine contraceptive devices (IUCDs) commonly used in India?

63. What medical conditions are considered contraindications for the use of intrauterine contraceptive devices (IUCDs) according to the medical eligibility criteria?

64. What are the additional medical applications and advantages of hormone-releasing intrauterine contraceptive devices (IUCDs) beyond contraception?

65. Provide a critical analysis of the World Health Organization's Medical Eligibility Criteria for the use of injectable medroxy-progesterone acetate as a contraceptive?

66. Provide information about Antra, an injectable contraceptive containing medroxyprogesterone acetate (MPA)?

67. What are the medical eligibility criteria established by the World Health Organization for the use of progesterone-only pills (POPs)?

68. Provide information about combined injectable contraceptives (CICs)?

69. Describe the transdermal contraceptive patch and its use as a contraceptive method?

70. What are the different methods available for female sterilization?

71. What are the criteria or guidelines for female sterilization procedures?

72. What are the various methods used for tubal ligation?

73. What are the factors contributing to the perception that male sterilization is simpler and safer compared to female sterilization?

74. What does NSV refer to in the context of sterilization procedures?

75. What key points would you like to address when counseling a couple considering vasectomy as a contraceptive option?

76. Provide a summary of the various methods used for tubal ligation?

77. What are the eligibility criteria established by the Government of India for female sterilization during a cesarean section?

78. What are the various techniques and timing options available for female tubal ligation?

79. What criteria are used to determine eligibility for female tubal ligation, and what preoperative assessments are typically conducted?

80. What is the Female Sterilization Insurance Scheme?

81. What benefits are associated with laparoscopic sterilization?

82. What are the potential long-term complications or effects of tubal ligation procedures?

83. What are the potential health advantages associated with tubal sterilization procedures?

84. What are the various techniques available for achieving female sterilization?

85. What are the potential complications or risks associated with tubal sterilization procedures?

86. What factors contribute to the failure of tubal sterilization procedures?

87. Explain the process of obtaining consent for tubal ligation procedures?

88. What are the situations where tubal recanalization procedures may be considered appropriate?

89. What factors contribute to the increased success of tubal recanalization procedures?

90. What considerations should be taken into account when prescribing contraceptives for a woman who is HIV positive?

91. What are the potential risks associated with undergoing a vasectomy procedure?
92. Provide an overview of contraceptive options available for women after childbirth?
93. What contraceptive options are included in the National Family Planning Programme of India?
94. What is postpartum intrauterine contraceptive device (PPIUCD) insertion?
95. What are the elements of the Family Planning Insurance Scheme (FPIS)?
96. Provide information on the usage, indications, benefits, and drawbacks of centchroman?
97. What initiatives and programs exist in India to address adolescent health, and what is their current status?
98. What are the reasons for utilizing contraception among adolescents, and what methods are available for them?
99. What advancements have been made in the field of male contraception in recent years?
100. Provide information about RISUG, also known as reversible inhibition of sperm under guidance?
101. How is non-scalpel vasectomy performed?
102. Explain what a female condom is and how it works?
103. What are the instructions for using a female condom, and what are its benefits?

GENETICS

1. Explain what chromosome microarray analysis is?
2. How is chromosome microarray analysis used in clinical practice?
3. What is preimplantation genetic testing, and what are the various methods employed for it?
4. What are the medical uses of preimplantation genetic testing?
5. What does pre-conception counseling entail?

6. How would you provide pre-conception counseling to a young woman with a history of a previous child with thalassemia major?
7. What is the purpose of preimplantation diagnostic techniques??
8. Provide information about Down syndrome?
9. What are the various screening methods available for detecting Down syndrome during pregnancy?
10. What is NIPT, and what is its current significance in prenatal screening?
11. What antenatal tests should be offered to a pregnant woman with a history of a previous child with Down syndrome, organized by trimester?
12. What are the considerations for antenatal monitoring in monochorionic twin pregnancies?
13. Explain what cell-free fetal DNA is?
14. What is the significance of cell-free fetal DNA screening in obstetric care?
15. What is involved in biochemical screening for Down syndrome?
16. What is the significance of fetal cell-free DNA in maternal blood?
17. Explain what pre-implantation genetic diagnosis (PGD) is?
18. Provide information about comprehensive chromosomal screening (CCS)?
19. What are the reasons for, advantages of, and potential drawbacks to PGD and CCS?
20. What factors increase the likelihood of neural tube defects?
21. What methods are used for screening for Down syndrome?
22. What options exist for pre-implantation genetic testing?
23. What does genetic counseling involve?
24. When should prenatal genetic counseling be offered, and to whom?
25. Explain what pre-implantation genetic diagnosis (PGD) is?
26. What are the indications for cell-free fetal DNA screening?
27. What are invasive prenatal diagnostic tests, and how are they used?
28. What qualities define a reliable screening test?

29. What are the screening procedures for detecting aneuploidies?
30. What is pre-implantation genetic diagnosis (PGD)?
31. What does genetic counseling involve?
32. In which patients is genetic counseling recommended?
33. What diagnostic procedures are available to assist in diagnosis?

Chapter - 7

MISCELLANEOUS

1. How is laser technology utilized in gynecology?
2. What are the circumstances that necessitate massive blood transfusion?
3. Provide information about the protocols for massive blood transfusion in obstetrics, including potential adverse reactions?
4. What are the foundational principles of collecting forensic evidence in cases involving sexual assault victims?
5. What is the POCSO Act, and what does it entail?
6. How is counseling typically provided to survivors of sexual assault?
7. How is PET-CT imaging utilized in the field of gynecology?
8. What are the ethical considerations surrounding uterine transplantation?
9. What criteria are used to select, evaluate, and screen patients for uterine transplantation?
10. What strategies can be implemented to enhance antenatal care amidst the COVID-19 pandemic?
11. How should suspected or confirmed cases of COVID-19 be managed during labor?
12. What steps would you take to care for a newborn born to a mother with suspected or confirmed COVID-19?
13. What is the definition of stem cells?
14. What potential applications does stem cell therapy have in obstetrics and gynecology?
15. How is MRI utilized in the field of obstetrics?
16. What are teratogens, and how do they affect pregnancy?

17. Explain viral teratogens and their impact?
18. What are the immune changes that occur during pregnancy?
19. What is the role of maternal immunization in protecting against various pathogens?
20. What does the PCPNDT Act entail?
21. What is the physiological basis of obesity?
22. How does obesity impact women's reproductive health?
23. What is NIPT, and how is it used in prenatal screening?
24. What is GeneXpert, and what are its applications?
25. What is foetal inflammatory response syndrome (FIRS), and what are its associated health complications?
26. What factors contribute to sudden intra-partum fetal demise, and how can counseling be provided in such cases?
27. What are the protocols for handling biological waste in the labor room?
28. What are universal precautions, and how are they applied in healthcare settings?
29. What is post-exposure prophylaxis, and when is it administered?
30. What are the potential consequences of Rubella infection on the fetus, and how can it be prevented?
31. What is known about the safety of vaccinations administered during pregnancy?
32. What are the key procedures involved in examining a survivor of sexual assault?
33. What is maternal near miss, and how is it defined?
34. What is obstetric audit, and how is it conducted?
35. What are the risk factors associated with hospital-acquired infections (HAIs), and what organisms commonly cause them?
36. What are the typical clinical manifestations of common hospital-acquired infections in obstetrics and gynecology?
37. What measures can be taken to prevent hospital-acquired infections?

38. What are the fundamental guidelines for collecting forensic evidence from a survivor of sexual assault?
39. How would you approach counseling for a woman who has experienced sexual assault?
40. What is the protocol for post-exposure prophylaxis against sexually transmitted infections and HIV in cases of sexual assault?
41. What is the method for calculating BMI, and what are the different BMI ranges?
42. How does BMI relate to obstetrics and gynecology?
43. What are the mechanisms involved in maintaining fluid and electrolyte balance after surgery?
44. What steps would you take to diagnose and address fluid and electrolyte imbalances following surgery?
45. What are the key principles underlying the functioning of obstetric high dependency units (HDUs)?
46. What steps would you take to establish a high dependency unit (HDU) in your hospital for obstetric care?
47. What is the Zika virus, and what are its characteristics?
48. What are the modes of transmission for the Zika virus?
49. What methods are used to diagnose Zika virus infection in pregnant women?
50. What are the potential effects of Zika virus infection on the fetus?
51. What are the considerations regarding the use of amniocentesis for diagnosing congenital Zika virus infection?
52. What are the indications for uterine transplant, its surgical procedure, ethical considerations, and factors contributing to transplant failure?
53. What viral infections are linked to congenital malformations?
54. What steps would you take to manage a case of dengue fever in a pregnant patient?
55. What are common areas of medical legal disputes in obstetrics?
56. What strategies can be implemented to minimize legal issues in obstetrics, considering both legal and ethical aspects?
57. What is necrotizing fasciitis, and how is it characterized?

58. What is involved in pre-conception counseling?
59. How would you counsel and manage a patient with a history of a neural tube defect in a previous child regarding her next pregnancy?
60. What are the potential complications associated with pregnancy in women of advanced maternal age?
61. How would you conduct screening and manage a patient of advanced maternal age?
62. How does domestic violence affect sexual and reproductive health?
63. What physiological and anatomical changes occur in the urinary system during pregnancy?
64. What is asymptomatic bacteriuria?
65. What impact does asymptomatic bacteriuria have on pregnancy?
66. What are the fundamental principles of caring for a survivor of sexual abuse?
67. What are the indicators used to measure bone turnover biochemically?
68. What methods are used to assess bone mineral density?
69. What treatments are available for managing osteoporosis?
70. How do implied consent and informed consent differ from each other?
71. What are some common areas of legal disputes in obstetrics?
72. What are the legal considerations surrounding birth asphyxia?
73. Provide a brief overview of the complications associated with blood transfusion?
74. What is stem cell banking, and what does it involve?
75. What are the fundamental principles guiding the collection of forensic evidence from a survivor of sexual assault?
76. How would you approach counseling for a woman who has experienced sexual assault?
77. Provide a brief overview of post-exposure prophylaxis (PEP) for HIV?
78. What are the essential considerations for establishing an adolescent health clinic in your hospital?

79. What are the risks to reproductive health faced by adolescent girls?
80. What preventive measures can be implemented through the clinic to mitigate reproductive health risks in adolescent girls?
81. What is the definition of micronutrients?
82. What roles do four specific micronutrients play in promoting maternal and fetal health?
83. What are the reasons for and methods of administering iron therapy to expectant fathers during pregnancy

SURGERIES

1. What measures can be taken to prevent ureteric injuries during endoscopic surgery?
2. Outline the approach to managing ureterovaginal fistula occurring after hysterectomy.
3. Compare and contrast the outcomes and considerations of total laparoscopic hysterectomy (TLH) versus non-descent vaginal hysterectomy (NDVH).
4. Categorize and provide concise descriptions of the different types of hysterectomy.
5. In what situations is ureteric injury more probable during surgery, and what preventive measures can be taken to minimize the risk?
6. What are the criteria and prerequisites for performing non-descent vaginal hysterectomy, and when is it typically indicated?
7. List the immediate and delayed post-operative complications associated with non-descent vaginal hysterectomy.
8. Detail the advantages and disadvantages of non-descent vaginal hysterectomy when compared to laparoscopic hysterectomy.

PROCEDURES

1. Discuss the indications for uterus transplant and explore its future prospects.
2. Examine the applications of umbilical cord banking and provide recommendations for its utilization.

3. Define fetal blood sampling and outline its indications.
4. Describe the potential sites for fetal blood sampling and discuss associated complications.
5. Explain chorionic villus sampling and detail its procedural method.
6. Explore the clinical uses and applications of chorionic villus sampling.
7. What are the characteristics and advancements associated with third-generation endometrial ablation techniques?
8. Compare and contrast the effectiveness of thermal endometrial ablation with levonorgestrel intrauterine system (IUS) for the management of menorrhagia.
9. Examine various interventional approaches used in treating benign gynecological conditions.
10. Discuss the technique and applications of uterine artery embolization.
11. Explain the procedure of uterine artery embolization.
12. List the indications for uterine artery embolization in modern obstetrics and gynecology.
13. Provide a concise overview of the techniques, benefits, and drawbacks associated with uterine artery embolization.
14. What are the clinical scenarios where chorionic villus sampling is indicated?
15. At what stage of pregnancy is chorionic villus sampling typically conducted?
16. What complications may arise from chorionic villus sampling, and what strategies are employed to manage them?
17. What genetic conditions or situations warrant the use of amniocentesis?
18. At what stage of pregnancy is amniocentesis typically recommended?
19. Examine the potential complications associated with amniocentesis and strategies for their prevention.

Chapter - 8

ONCOLOGY

1. Explain various approaches to screening for cervical cancer.
2. Discuss the factors contributing to the development of cervical cancer and outline strategies for preventing it.
3. Explain the contemporary recommendations for screening for cervical cancer.
4. Detail the strategies for addressing precancerous cervical lesions.
5. Enumerate different methods used to screen for cervical cancer.
6. Discuss the Human Papillomavirus (HPV) vaccine and its role in preventing cervical cancer.
7. Explore the utilization of liquid-based cytology as a technique in cervical cancer screening.
8. Examine the current recommendations for cervical cancer screening.
9. What are the benefits associated with liquid-based cytology compared to conventional Pap smears?
10. Describe the mechanism behind prolonged Human Papillomavirus (HPV) infection in the cervix and its clinical implications.
11. Explain methods for detecting Human Papillomavirus (HPV) infection and strategies for its prevention.
12. What are the updated recommendations for cervical cancer screening?
13. Examine the significance of Pap smear and HPV testing in the screening process for cervical cancer.
14. What benefits does liquid-based cytology offer compared to traditional Pap smear methods?

15. Examine the importance of HPV DNA testing in cervical cancer screening.

16. Outline the recommended clinical pathway for managing Low-Grade Squamous Intraepithelial Lesions (LSIL) in a 36-year-old female.

17. Provide an overview of colposcopic evaluation techniques for cervical intraepithelial neoplasia.

18. What are the four primary features that clinicians typically assess during colposcopic examination to diagnose cervical intraepithelial neoplasia?

19. What are the characteristic appearances of lesions in both low-grade and high-grade cervical intraepithelial neoplasia after the application of normal saline, 5% acetic acid solution, and Lugol's iodine solution during colposcopic examination?

20. What is the Reid Colposcopic Index, and how does it contribute to the assessment of cervical lesions during colposcopy?

21. What are the key diagnostic considerations for cervical intraepithelial neoplasia?

22. What are the methods used for early detection of cervical cancer through screening?

23. What are the benefits associated with liquid-based cytology compared to traditional Pap smear methods?

24. What are the mechanisms underlying persistent human papillomavirus (HPV) infection in the cervix, and what is its clinical significance?

25. What are the diagnostic methods for detecting human papillomavirus (HPV) infection, and what strategies can be employed for its prevention?

26. What are some contemporary approaches to screening for premalignant cervical lesions?

27. What are the criteria for recommending colposcopy, and how are the findings interpreted?

28. What is the role of Loop Electrosurgical Excision Procedure (LEEP) in managing premalignant cervical lesions?

29. What are the appropriate management steps for a 60-year-old woman presenting with malodorous vaginal discharge and postcoital bleeding?

30. What are the staging criteria utilized by the International Federation of Gynecology and Obstetrics (FIGO) to categorize cervical cancer?

31. What are the various methods employed for staging cervical cancer?

32. What factors influence the prognosis of cervical cancer?

33. What are the recommended treatment approaches for cervical cancer diagnosed at stage IB?

34. What is radical trachelectomy and how is it utilized in the management of cervical cancer?

35. What are the factors that increase the risk of developing cervical cancer?

36. What are the available treatment options for cervical intraepithelial neoplasia?

37. What is the transformation zone of the cervix, and how is it assessed during evaluation?

38. What are the current recommendations for cervical cancer screening?

39. How does the lymphatic drainage pattern of the cervix influence surgical planning and treatment decisions?

40. Outline the clinical manifestations of cervical cancer, particularly at stage IB, in a woman aged 31.

41. What are the potential benefits of surgical treatment compared to radiotherapy, or vice versa, for managing cervical cancer in a patient like this?

42. What are the key aspects of the HPV vaccine?

43. What are the mechanisms by which human papillomavirus (HPV) contributes to the development of cervical cancer?

44. How does the detection of HPV contribute to cervical cancer screening and follow-up?

45. What are the key aspects of vaccines targeting human papillomavirus (HPV)?

46. What are the available therapeutic approaches for managing cervical intraepithelial neoplasia (CIN)?
47. What is the pathophysiology of Human Papillomavirus (HPV) infection, and how does it lead to the development of cancer?
48. What are the typical progression patterns of Human Papillomavirus (HPV) infections?
49. What are the methods used to diagnose Human Papillomavirus (HPV) infection?
50. What are the perspectives regarding HPV vaccination?
51. How does genetic counseling impact the management of ovarian cancer?
52. What is a hormonally active ovarian tumor?
53. What are the different pathological types associated with it?
54. What are the diagnostic methods and treatment strategies for ovarian tumors that secrete estrogen?
55. What are the indications that may lead to suspicion of hereditary breast/ovarian cancer syndrome?
56. What preventive measures can be taken for individuals with a family history of ovarian cancer?
57. What are the most recent staging criteria for ovarian cancer according to the International Federation of Gynecology and Obstetrics (FIGO)?
58. What treatment options would you consider for a 55-year-old woman diagnosed with stage III epithelial ovarian cancer?
59. What are the components of the FIGO classification system for ovarian carcinoma?
60. What are the various conditions that can mimic ovarian tumors, leading to differential diagnoses?
61. What are the molecular mechanisms underlying ovarian cancer, and how do they influence clinical management?
62. What treatment options would you consider for managing a unilateral solid ovarian tumor in a 17-year-old girl?
63. What are the categories used to classify benign ovarian tumors?

64. What are the diagnostic approaches, potential complications, and treatment strategies for benign cystic teratomas?
65. What are the markers used in the diagnosis or monitoring of ovarian tumors?
66. How do ovarian tumor markers contribute to the management of ovarian cancer?
67. What factors increase the likelihood of developing ovarian carcinoma?
68. What is the latest research indicating regarding the effectiveness of screening for ovarian carcinoma?
69. What are the key principles guiding the management of advanced-stage ovarian carcinoma?
70. How would you approach the treatment of ovarian malignancy in a 23-year-old woman?
71. What are the potential causes of an adnexal mass in a 19-year-old unmarried woman?
72. What diagnostic tests or procedures would you consider for evaluating the adnexal mass in the 19-year-old unmarried woman?
73. What are the fundamental principles guiding the management of germ cell tumors?
74. What does chemoprophylaxis entail in the context of ovarian cancer?
75. What are the indications for bilateral salpingectomy?
76. What are the indications for peritoneal stripping in cases of peritoneal carcinoma?
77. What are ovarian germ cell tumors?
78. How is dysgerminoma typically managed?
79. What are the biomarkers associated with gynecological cancers?
80. What is the role of intraperitoneal chemotherapy in managing ovarian cancer?
81. What are the strategies for reducing the risk of developing epithelial ovarian cancer?
82. What is the role of fertility-sparing surgery in the management of ovarian malignancies?

83. What are the different categories of malignant ovarian tumors arising from germ cells?
84. What is hereditary breast and ovarian cancer syndrome?
85. What is the Risk of Malignancy Index (RMI) used for in assessing ovarian masses?
86. What is meant by adjuvant chemotherapy in cancer treatment?
87. What treatment options would you consider for a patient diagnosed with malignant epithelial ovarian tumor?
88. What are the different types of ovarian tumors arising from germ cells?
89. What are the typical laboratory and radiological findings, as well as the management approach, for dysgerminoma?
90. What is familial ovarian cancer syndrome, and what are its characteristics?
91. How do proteomic and genomic techniques contribute to the diagnosis of ovarian cancer?
92. What are the indications for prophylactic oophorectomy?
93. What are the considerations for utilizing conservative surgery in the management of gynecological malignancies?
94. What are the surgical procedures and techniques available for preserving fertility in ovarian and cervical cancers?
95. What are the possible differential diagnoses for an adnexal mass in a young woman?
96. What are the criteria for selecting fertility-sparing surgery and the follow-up protocols for a young woman diagnosed with a malignant ovarian tumor?
97. What diagnostic considerations arise when a 13-year-old girl presents with a unilateral adnexal mass?
98. What are the possible differential diagnoses for a unilateral adnexal mass in a 13-year-old girl?
99. What treatment approach would you consider for managing a germ cell tumor in this girl?
100. What are the various types of ovarian tumors that can occur in adolescent girls?

101. What are the typical clinical features associated with malignant ovarian tumors?

102. What types of tumors are commonly associated with ovarian malignancies?

103. What is the role of neoadjuvant chemotherapy in the treatment of ovarian malignancies, and how does it impact patient outcomes?

104. How about detailing the recent updates or changes to the FIGO staging system for endometrial cancer instead?

105. Explore the key prognostic factors and molecular markers that influence the treatment and outcome of endometrial cancer?

106. How endometrial carcinoma is classified according to the latest FIGO system?

107. Explore the methods and strategies for diagnosing premalignant and malignant endometrial lesions in women?

108. Discuss the approaches for identifying and treating endometrial intraepithelial neoplasia?

109. Explain the causes and potential complications of endometrial hyperplasia?

110. What are the recommended treatment options for managing simple cystic hyperplasia in a perimenopausal woman?

111. What diagnostic steps should be taken for a 61-year-old woman experiencing post-menopausal bleeding?

112. What are the possible conditions that could present with post-menopausal bleeding, and how can they be differentiated?

113. What diagnostic tests and examinations would you recommend for evaluating the patient's post-menopausal bleeding?

114. What are the key approaches to treating endometrial carcinoma?

115. What are the potential underlying factors contributing to postmenopausal vaginal bleeding in a 53-year-old woman?

116. Outline a systematic approach for diagnosing and treating postmenopausal vaginal bleeding in a 53-year-old woman?

117. What are the recommended clinical protocols for managing stage I adenocarcinoma of the uterine body according to current guidelines?

118. Explain the condition known as endometrial hyperplasia.
119. Categorize endometrial hyperplasia types based on their risk for developing into malignancy?
120. What are the fundamental approaches to treating atypical hyperplasia?
121. How is chemotherapy utilized in the treatment of endometrial cancer?
122. What is the significance of lymphadenectomy in the treatment plan for endometrial cancer?
123. What diagnostic steps would you take when evaluating post-menopausal bleeding?
124. What are the components and stages of the FIGO classification system used for endometrial carcinoma?
125. What steps would you take to assess and manage postmenopausal bleeding in a 54-year-old woman?
126. What clinical assessments would you conduct for a 54-year-old woman presenting with postmenopausal bleeding?
127. What diagnostic tests would you recommend for further evaluation of postmenopausal bleeding in this patient?
128. What are the recommended management strategies for treating endometrial carcinoma in this patient?
129. What are the potential causes of galactorrhea in women who are not breastfeeding?
130. What diagnostic steps would you take and what treatment options would you consider for a 33-year-old woman who has been experiencing unilateral breast discharge for the past 6 months, and has given birth at least once?
131. What are the histological subtypes of vaginal intraepithelial neoplasia (VaIN)?
132. What are the various approaches to treating vaginal intraepithelial neoplasia (VaIN)?
133. Provide information on vaginal intraepithelial neoplasia (VaIN), including its characteristics and implications?
134. What is the role of sentinel lymph node biopsy in the management of vulvar cancer?

135. What are the potential etiologies and treatment options for recurrent ulcers in the vulvar region?

136. Provide an overview of vulvar intraepithelial neoplasia (VIN), including its characteristics and implications?

137. What are the considerations regarding lymph node management during radical vulvectomy procedures?

138. Explain the concept of sentinel lymph nodes?

139. What is the significance of sentinel lymph node biopsy in the treatment of gynecological cancers?

140. How is PET-CT imaging utilized in the field of gynecology?

141. What are the different methods of preserving fertility in female cancer patients?

142. Provide an overview of the applications of PET-CT imaging in the context of gynecological malignancies?

143. Provide a summary of the combined chemotherapy and radiation therapy approach for the treatment of cervical cancer?

144. Provide a concise explanation of the clinical utility of serum CA 125 levels as a tumor marker?

145. What are the principles and indications for selective pelvic lymphadenectomy in the context of gynecologic malignancies?

146. What is the rationale behind the use of concurrent chemoradiation and how is it employed in the management of gynecological cancers?

147. What are some examples of tumor markers commonly utilized in the field of gynecology?

148. Elaborate on the clinical relevance of different tumor markers used in gynecological conditions?

149. Could you provide an overview of the classification of gestational trophoblastic diseases (GTD) and their pathogenesis?

150. What are the recommended management approaches for a patient diagnosed with a hydatidiform mole (H.mole) alongside a coexisting live fetus at 14 weeks of gestation?

151. How would you approach the case of a 37-year-old woman, who is a mother of three, presenting with irregular vaginal bleeding?

She has a history of a molar pregnancy 8 months ago, her serum beta HCG is 12000 mIU/ml, ultrasound reveals a theca lutein cyst measuring 6 x 6 cm, and a chest X-ray shows two coin-shaped lesions.

152. What is the FIGO staging and risk assessment for the described clinical scenario?
153. What treatment options would you consider for managing the described clinical case?
154. What are the diagnostic methods used to identify trophoblastic disease?
155. What are the approaches to managing trophoblastic disease?
156. What are the histological classifications used for categorizing gestational trophoblastic neoplasia (GTN)?
157. How would you conduct a diagnostic evaluation for a suspected case of gestational trophoblastic neoplasia (GTN)?
158. What treatment options are available for managing low-risk gestational trophoblastic neoplasia (GTN)?
159. What are the different types of gestational trophoblastic neoplasia (GTN)?
160. What are the staging criteria for gestational trophoblastic neoplasia (GTN) and the modified WHO prognostic scoring system?
161. What are the common signs and symptoms associated with gestational trophoblastic neoplasia (GTN)?
162. Explain the World Health Organization (WHO) risk scoring system used in gestational trophoblastic neoplasia (GTN)?
163. What are the single-agent and multi-agent chemotherapy regimens used in the treatment of gestational trophoblastic neoplasia (GTN), and what is the recommended follow-up protocol?

Chapter - 9

ANATOMY AND PHYSIOLOGY

1. What are the different anatomical classifications of the female pelvis?
2. What obstetrical implications do the anatomical variations of the female pelvis have, and how do they affect the progress of labor?
3. Explain the lymphatic drainage patterns of the female genital tract?
4. What is the significance of lymphadenectomy in the management of genital malignancies?
5. What are the branches of the anterior and posterior divisions of the internal iliac artery?
6. Provide a concise overview of the procedure for internal iliac artery embolization and its indications?
7. Outline the path of the ureter from its point of origin to its insertion into the bladder?
8. What are the common locations where ureteral injuries may occur during surgical procedures?
9. What are some strategies for preventing ureteral injuries during surgery, and how would you approach the management of accidental ureteral ligation during suturing?
10. What are the anatomical features of the internal iliac artery, and how does its anatomy relate to clinical considerations in obstetrics and gynecology?
11. Explain the contents and significance of the superficial perineal pouch?
12. Describe the path of the pudendal nerve, particularly in the context of administering a pudendal block?
13. What structures comprise the anatomy of the perineum?

14. What are the classifications of obstetric injuries to the anal sphincter?
15. What are the approaches to managing a third-degree perineal injury?
16. Describe the structure and components of the pelvic diaphragm?
17. Explain the Pelvic Organ Prolapse Quantification (POP-Q) system as it relates to uterine and vaginal vault prolapse?
18. Describe the embryological development of the vagina, preferably with a diagram?
19. What are some examples of anatomical abnormalities that can result in primary congenital anomalies?
20. What are the surgical options available for managing congenital abnormalities of the Müllerian duct in cases of primary amenorrhea?
21. Discuss the anatomical features relevant to surgical procedures involving the urinary bladder?
22. What measures can be taken to minimize the risk of bladder injury during obstetric and gynecological surgeries?
23. What methods can be used to detect bladder injury during or after surgery, and what are the appropriate steps for managing it?
24. What are the sources of blood supply to the female reproductive organs?
25. What are the indications for uterine artery embolization in obstetrics and gynecology, and how does it contribute to patient management?
26. What are some potential complications that can arise from uterine artery embolization?
27. Provide an overview of the anatomical structures comprising the anterior abdominal wall?
28. What are the various types of surgical incisions commonly employed in gynecological procedures?
29. What are the anatomical considerations relevant to pelvic organ support?
30. What are the causes of uterine and vaginal vault prolapse in nulliparous women, and what surgical approaches can be considered for their management?
31. What role does the uterosacral ligament play in gynecological conditions and procedures?

32. What are the anatomical features of the female perineum, and how do they relate to obstetrics?

33. Discuss the vascular anatomy of the anterior abdominal wall with respect to the placement of surgical ports?

34. What are some potential complications associated with entry during laparoscopic surgery?

35. Provide an overview of the structural anatomy and physiological function of the anal sphincter complex?

36. What are the risk factors for anorectal injury during childbirth, and could you discuss the evolving perspective on episiotomy?

37. Explain the surgical anatomy of the cervix and its lymphatic drainage?

38. What options are available for preserving fertility in patients diagnosed with cervical cancer?

39. What is the rationale behind combining chemotherapy and radiation therapy, and how is this approach applied in the treatment of cervical cancer?

40. Describe the path taken by the ureter in the body?

41. What are the potential sites of injury or damage to the ureter during obstetric and gynecological surgeries?

42. What are the methods used to diagnose ureteral injury, and what approaches are employed for its management?

43. What are the different retroperitoneal spaces within the pelvis, and what are their defining boundaries?

44. How do the pelvic retroperitoneal spaces play a role in gynecological conditions and procedures?

45. Explain the structures that support the uterus and discuss issues related to posterior compartment defects?

46. What are the blood supply, lymphatic drainage, and nerve innervation of the cervix, and how do these anatomical features relate to clinical considerations?

47. Provide an overview of the anatomical features of the ureter within the pelvis?

48. Where are the potential locations for ureteric injury during pelvic surgical procedures?

49. What measures can be taken to reduce the risk of ureteric injuries during pelvic surgery?
50. What are the principal blood vessels that provide blood supply to the pelvic region?
51. What is the clinical importance of the collateral circulation in the pelvis, particularly in the context of internal iliac artery ligation?
52. What are some potential adverse outcomes associated with internal iliac artery ligation?
53. What are the structural characteristics of the placenta?
54. What are some of the anomalies that can occur during the development of the placenta?
55. What are the potential complications associated with placenta accreta, increta, and percreta?

PHYSIOLOGY

1. How does normal placentation occur?
2. What are the consequences of abnormal placentation?
3. How does the physiology of lactation work?
4. How should a new mother who is unable to initiate lactation be managed?
5. What are the physiological changes in coagulation that occur during pregnancy?
6. What are the risk factors for thrombosis during pregnancy, and what methods should be considered for thromboprophylaxis?
7. How is the volume of amniotic fluid regulated physiologically?
8. How does circulation occur within the placenta?
9. How does renal physiology change during pregnancy?
10. How does the corpus luteum function and what is its role?
11. What are the implications of corpus luteum dysfunction?
12. How is amniotic fluid formed physiologically?
13. What are the physiological functions of amniotic fluid?

14. What are the clinical consequences of abnormalities in amniotic fluid?
15. What changes occur in the urinary tract during pregnancy?
16. How does the implantation of a pregnancy occur?
17. What placental abnormalities are associated with abnormal placentation?
18. What is the process of wound healing?
19. How can the risk of dehiscence in a Caesarean scar be minimized?
20. How does the physiological process of ovulation occur?
21. How does the corpus luteum develop?
22. How do blood parameters alter during pregnancy?
23. How are the physiological changes in blood during pregnancy related to the development of anemia?
24. Explain the circulatory dynamics of the placenta.
25. What are the factors or conditions that can disrupt placental circulation?
26. Detail the process of Graafian follicle development and ovulation.
27. What is the role of the corpus luteum in the reproductive cycle?
28. How is corpus luteum deficiency diagnosed and treated?
29. What are the typical breast changes experienced by first-time pregnant women?
30. What are the usual breast issues that arise during pregnancy and postpartum, and how are they treated?
31. Describe the process of placental formation.
32. Explain how fetal circulation is affected by the diaphragm.
33. Detail the process of milk ejection in lactating individuals.
34. What does early initiation of breastfeeding involve?
35. How can successful breastfeeding be encouraged?
36. What are the various types of skin changes that can occur during pregnancy?
37. What are the different reasons for itching during pregnancy?

38. What are the strategies for treating pruritus associated with pregnancy?
39. How does thyroid function typically change during pregnancy?
40. What are the risks linked to hypothyroidism during pregnancy?
41. What are the signs of postpartum thyroiditis, and how can it be treated?
42. What are the natural alterations in the vagina throughout the menstrual cycle?
43. What methods are used to identify bacterial vaginosis?
44. Explain the syndromic approach used to manage cases involving vaginal discharge?
45. Detail the hormonal processes involved in ovulation.
46. What are the different methods available for evaluating ovulation?
47. What is the significance of human chorionic gonadotropin (hCG) levels in early pregnancy?
48. How is a missed abortion typically managed in the first trimester?
49. What are the alterations seen in the liver and biliary system during pregnancy?
50. What are the clinical signs and laboratory indicators of intrahepatic cholestasis of pregnancy (ICP)?
51. What are the potential risks to the fetus and newborn associated with intrahepatic cholestasis of pregnancy, and what measures can be taken to mitigate them?
52. How does the coagulation system function change throughout pregnancy?
53. What is the mechanism underlying disseminated intravascular coagulation (DIC)?
54. What are the considerations for blood transfusion and component therapy in patients with DIC?
55. Describe the fetal circulation using a diagram?
56. What are the typical serum levels for FSH, LH, estradiol (E2), progesterone, and testosterone?

57. Why is it important to monitor these hormones in gynecological care?
58. What hormones does the placenta produce?
59. What are some of the disorders or conditions affecting the placenta?
60. What types of disorders affect placental blood flow?
61. What roles does follicle-stimulating hormone (FSH) play in the body?
62. When are gonadotropins typically prescribed in gynecological practice?
63. What are some common medications used to inhibit gonadotropin activity?
64. How does the thyroid gland typically change during pregnancy?
65. What are the roles of the fetal thyroid gland?
66. Why is it important to routinely screen for thyroid function during pregnancy?
67. What are the distinct stages of the ovarian cycle?
68. Describe the stages involved in the development and differentiation of ovarian follicles.
69. What factors contribute to the process of ovulation?
70. What does the pathological assessment of the placenta involve
71. Could you elaborate on various types of placental abnormalities and their implications?
72. Explain the circulation system in the fetus?
73. How are Inhibin A and B utilized in obstetrics and gynecology?
74. What are the typical alterations in serum beta-hCG levels during a healthy pregnancy?
75. What are the reasons for evaluating beta-hCG levels during pregnancy, and what clinical insights do they provide?
76. What are the signs of normal ovulation?
77. What are the methods used to test for ovulation?
78. What are the fundamental principles underlying controlled ovarian hyperstimulation?

79. How does the body naturally produce amniotic fluid?
80. Provide a labeled diagram of a Graafian follicle?
81. What are the methods used to assess ovarian reserve, and how should the results of each test be interpreted?
82. What are the available treatment options for women with diminished ovarian reserve, assuming other fertility factors are normal?

EMBRYOLOGY

1. Provide an overview of the embryological development of the female reproductive tract?
2. What are the methods used to diagnose and treat bicornuate uterus?
3. Describe the stages of human embryo development.
4. What key factors are involved in sexual differentiation during development?
5. What are some substances known to cause birth defects in developing embryos?
6. Describe the formation and composition of the umbilical cord?
7. What are the different types of umbilical cord abnormalities, and why are they clinically significant?